Advance praise for *Why Retire? Career Strategies for Third Age Nurses*

"This wonderful book characterizes the saying "We aren't getting older. We are getting wiser and better!" Now and in the foreseeable future, our ability to improve the health of individuals and communities is dependent upon the availability of a qualified, experienced workforce. The nation needs nurses in their Third Age in a variety of roles to assist with the burgeoning growth of novice nurses. This book explores the possibilities that exist for nurses to continue their work in human caring. It is a must-read for nurses who are considering retirement."

–Linda Burnes Bolton, DrPH, RN, FAAN
Vice President and Chief Nursing Officer,
Cedars-Sinai Medical Center
Los Angeles, California

"In Why Retire? Career Strategies for Third Age Nurses, Fay Bower and William A. Sadler present a powerful vision for individual and social renewal—one capable of revitalizing the health care workforce and enhancing the well-being and financial security of an entire generation of nurses. They couple this perspective with a compelling blueprint for realizing these ideas in ways both practical and timely. This book is essential reading for anyone interested in realizing the vast opportunity present in the aging of the baby boomers."

Founder/CEC
Author, *Encore: I*
Matters in the Se.....

D1275402

"This beautiful book is a must-have for everyone to create a life of significance for the Third Age and beyond. You will be transformed by a personal journey of envisioning possibilities and intentionally executing your idealized professional and personal future for the second half of your life. Enjoy the transformation!"

–Karlene M. Kerfoot, PhD, RN, NEA-BC, FAAN
Vice President and Chief Clinical Officer
Aurora Health Care
Milwaukee, Wisconsin

"This book will be especially helpful to nurse leaders seeking ways to extend the work life of experienced nurses nearing the traditional retirement stage of their career. Organizational examples help establish a new work paradigm for these valuable members of the nursing workforce. Using the six principles of the Third Age years, the authors provide a positive approach to aging and how Third Age nurses might reinvent themselves to continue a satisfying career that remains central to the caring profession of nursing."

–Joyce C. Clifford, PhD, RN, FAAN
President and CEO
The Institute for Nursing Healthcare Leadership

why retire?

Career Strategies for
Third Age Nurses

By Fay L. Bower, DNSc, FAAN, and
William A. Sadler, PhD

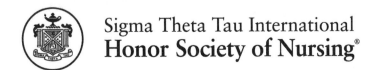

Sigma Theta Tau International
Honor Society of Nursing®

Sigma Theta Tau International

Publisher: Renee Wilmeth
Acquisitions Editor: Cynthia Saver, RN, MS
Project Editor: Carla Hall
Copy Editor: Kevin Kent
Proofreader: Jacqueline E. Tirey
Indexer: Jane Palmer

Cover Design by: Gary Adair
Interior Design and Page Composition by: Rebecca Harmon

Printed in the United States of America
Printing and Binding by Edwards Brothers, Inc.

Sigma Theta Tau International
550 West North Street
Indianapolis, IN 46202

To order additional books, buy in bulk, or order for corporate use, contact Nursing Knowledge International at 888.NKI.4YOU (888.654.4968/U.S. and Canada) or +1.317.634.8171 (outside U.S. and Canada).

To request a review copy for course adoption, e-mail solutions@nursingknowledge.org, or contact Cindy Jo Everett directly at 888.NKI.4YOU (888.654.4968/U.S. and Canada) or +1.317.917.4983 (outside U.S. and Canada).

To request author information, or for speaker or other media requests, contact Rachael McLaughlin of the Honor Society of Nursing, Sigma Theta Tau International, at 888.634.7575 (U.S. and Canada) or +1.317.634.8171 (outside U.S. and Canada).

ISBN-13: 9781-930538-76-4

Library of Congress Cataloging-in-Publication Data

Bower, Fay Louise.
  Why retire? : career strategies for third-age nurses / by Fay L. Bower
and William Sadler.
      p. ; cm.
  Includes bibliographical references.
  ISBN 978-1-930538-76-4
1. Nurses--Retirement. 2. Nursing--Practice. I. Sadler, William
Alan. II. Sigma Theta Tau International. III. Title.
  [DNLM: 1. Middle Aged--psychology. 2. Nurses--supply & distribution.
3. Personnel Management. 4. Retirement. WY 77 B786w 2009]
  RT86.7.B685 2009
  610.73068--dc22
                                    2009010280
First Printing
2009

Dedication

To all of those I have had the pleasure of teaching and working with, for without these opportunities I would not have been able to sustain interest and energy in nursing and education for more than 50 years. Their individual and collective accomplishments are, in part, what makes my professional life worthwhile.

–Fay Bower

In memory of Emre Edepli, a beloved grandson whose too-short life enriched our lives immensely.

–Bill Sadler

Acknowledgements

The authors wish to thank the countless nurses who have shared with us their insights, views, experiences, hopes, and concerns, without which this book could not have been written. In addition, we want to thank many individuals who have given generously of their time and knowledge about specific areas, in particular:

Marcia Canton

Linda Clever

Nancy Collins

Kathryn Hanson

Barbara Hatcher

James Krefft

Anna Mullins

Patricia Reineke

Andrea Segura

Maria Vezina

Steve Carpowich

Ed Coakley

Martha Giggleman

Kathy Harris

Kathryn Johnson

Terry Lowd

Lisa Ohmstede

Cindy Steckel

Jennifer Vallance

About the Authors

Fay L. Bower, DNSc, FAAN

Fay L. Bower has been practicing nursing for nearly 60 years and has been a nurse leader for almost that entire time. She has a BSN, a master's, and a doctorate—the latter earned at the University of California. Since the mid-1960s, the focus of her career has been on educating nurses and nurse leaders. Currently, she is chair of the Department of Nursing at Holy Names University in Oakland, California, where she has spearheaded the Third Age nurse initiatives, including the formation of the Center for Third Age Nurses at Holy Names. Prior to that, she was president of Clarkson College, vice president of academic affairs and dean of the School of Nursing at the University of San Francisco, and dean of the School of Nursing at San Jose State University.

Throughout her career, Bower has been elected to serve at the highest leadership levels within many organizations and associations. Her family keeps her both grounded and energized for all the work she does.

William A. Sadler, PhD

Since receiving his doctorate from Harvard University, William A. Sadler has been a professor, senior administrator, author, consultant, community leader, and noted speaker at local, national, and international conferences. He is the author of six books, and his book *The Third Age: Six Principles of Growth and Renewal After Forty* led to the formation of The Center for Third Age Leadership. Translated into several languages, it was selected by the Korean Broadcast System for one of its 2006 Book of the Week programs. His newest book, *Changing Course: Navigating Life After Fifty*, with co-author James Krefft, PhD, is based on 20 years of research.

Sadler is professor of sociology and business at Holy Names University in Oakland, California, where he teaches MBA leadership courses. He has been teaching at Holy Names for 20 years. Co-founder and director of research for The Center for Third Age Leadership, he and his wife, Sallie, split their residences between Oakland and the Maine coast.

TABLE OF CONTENTS

Foreword

The numbers are daunting: The projected RN shortage in the United States could be as high as 500,000 by 2025. At its core, the shortage will be driven by the inability to replace the large number of RNs born in the baby boomer generation who are expected to retire from the nursing workforce during the next 15 years. As nurses, we live the impact of a nurse shortage on a daily basis and understand better than most the implications of losing tens of thousands of experienced nurses to retirement. Part of this loss, it turns out, can be attributed to a cultural view of aging as a time to retire from the workforce.

Fortunately, a new paradigm on aging has emerged from William A. Sadler, PhD, co-author of *Why Retire?* Termed the *Third Age,* the period of life stretching from 50 to 75 years has shed its negative reputation as a period of decline, disuse, and disease and has been transformed into a positive, energizing time for renewal and growth.

Sadler tosses out old models of aging and declares that the most important challenge for those in the Third Age is "learning to tap their creative potential to sustain second growth, allowing them to experience fulfillment and make a difference in the world."

I couldn't agree more. These words will resonate with nurses, as they did with Fay Bower, DNSc, FAAN, Sadler's co-author. A tireless Third-Ager herself who has retired "unsuccessfully" several times, Bower collaborated with Sadler to apply Third Age concepts to nurses through her work at Holy Names University, ultimately creating the Center for Third Age Nurses along the way. Bower's experiences with senior nurses complement Sadler's findings. What they have found is that nurses 50 and older still love nursing and want to contribute to the health care profession, but too many feel burned out and are unaware of options that can allow them to remain in nursing without the physical difficulties. Fortunately, *Why Retire?* offers these Third Age nurses a way to rethink, remap, and renew their careers during their next stage of life.

In essence, this book speaks effectively on three levels.

- Nurses younger than 50 can integrate the principles into future career plans.
- Nurses already in the Third Age will find a wealth of wisdom and strategies for getting the most out of this important time in their lives.
- Health care leaders and executives will find *Why Retire?* an essential guidebook to be included in their toolbox of resources for dealing with the nursing shortage.

That last group is particularly key from a societal perspective. Patients need—and deserve—qualified nurses in all levels and positions of health care, from bedside to executive. By tapping into the expertise of Third Age nurses, administrators have an incredible advantage in dealing with the nursing shortage crisis. Nurse experts can transfer their knowledge to younger practitioners, who reap the benefits of experience, grace, and an innate intuition of what works and what nurses need to do their jobs with joy and satisfaction.

Fortunately, *Why Retire?* is a practical book. The authors use straightforward exercises and nurse-specific examples to illustrate their points. Chapters include information on how nurses can rethink retirement, strategies to help them redirect their careers, and how hospitals can more effectively retain senior nurses. The book concludes with strategies for creating the nurse workforce of tomorrow.

Every now and then a book comes along whose insights and ideas change our perspective about how we see our lives and the opportunities before us. Enjoy *Why Retire?* and discover new meaning and how you may continue to enjoy all that is good from the nursing profession.

–Peter I. Buerhaus, PhD, RN, FAAN
Valere Potter Professor of Nursing
Director, Center for Interdisciplinary Health Workforce Studies
Institute for Medicine and Public Heath
Vanderbilt University Medical Center
Nashville, Tennessee, USA

Introduction

Health care has always been an important concern for American people; recently, it has become a dominant national issue. Many questions have been raised, discussed, and debated about its costs, quality, accessibility, viability, extent of coverage, and future modes of delivery. However, one issue that has not received nearly enough attention is the current shortage of nurses. Today, health care is threatened by a shrinking number of nurses to provide the care our population needs. Recent projections estimate this shortage will continue and reach somewhere between half a million and 1 million nurses in less than a decade (Buerhaus, 2008). The shortage has already reached critical proportions and will only be exacerbated by demographics, with the number of aged patients in the United States predicted to expand exponentially. The combination of many more people needing health care and far fewer professionals providing the care creates a situation that needs immediate and concerted attention.

Health care organizations of all kinds have implemented several strategies to address this shortage, but to date none of these strategies has resolved the problem for a variety of reasons. Recruitment of new nurses for nursing schools is certainly one obvious strategy, but nursing schools are not able to handle vast numbers of new students. Even if they were, the baby boomers, who currently fill the ranks of nurses, are a much larger group than the next cohort; in short, the younger generation doesn't have enough people to take the places of baby boomers who are retiring. Some nursing schools have initiated accelerated programs to prepare nurses faster, but speed runs the risk of inadequate preparation for an increasingly complex and demanding role. A high turnover rate of new nurses suggests this approach generates its own problems and does not adequately address the need for a sustained cadre of highly committed, properly educated nurses.

Other strategies have been tried, with poor or problematic results. Travel nurses and foreign nurses have been recruited as a way to attract experienced nurses during the nurse shortage. Bonuses have been offered as another method for attracting seasoned and experienced nurses. All three options have had their problems and have not been able to reduce the nurse shortage. Travel nurses often do not stay beyond their contracted time frame, and while in the job, they often have a problem with commitment to the agency. Foreign nurses must face changes in cultural expectations and language; patients are often frightened by their approach and perceive they are not understood. Bonuses are a great recruitment strategy but have not worked as a retention strategy. As soon as the time frame for the bonus is over, nurses leave for another bonus. Also, nurses who receive bonuses often have conflicts with other nurses in the same position who did not get a bonus.

Another strategic option to stem the tide of the nurse shortage is the subject of this book. That strategy is to retain senior nurses in health care, especially nurses approaching retirement age who are still healthy, vital, and open to the possibility of continuing to function in health care in a new or different way. Recent surveys of senior nurses, such as those conducted for the Center for Third Age Nurses (NurseWeek, 2008), have found many of them are interested in postponing or redefining retirement if they can practice nursing in ways more compatible to their interests and needs, both personal and economic. These nurses represent an invaluable resource to health care and our society. Given the positive changes within an aging workforce, people who previously were expected to retire into leisured "golden years" are increasingly being recognized as invaluable resources to society, the economy, and their professions.

Furthermore, changes in the economy are pressuring individuals to continue working to meet expenses and expand investments and savings to sustain them in old age. Already, fewer nurses are seeking what has been labeled retirement; many are questioning the desirability of a retired lifestyle, with its implication of sitting back and doing nothing. An important aspect of retirement is the fact that the general population—and this includes nurses—is growing older and is in better health than ever. These people need to remain active, engaged, and involved in meaningful endeavors to fulfill the second half of life.

Research into the dramatic changes in the life course, particularly the years after 50, has suggested newer and more effective ways to manage the later years of life. Many senior nurses are open to an alternative to conventional retirement—changing direction rather than pulling themselves out of the action. These nurses represent a sizable population who can be recruited to stay in nursing and meet the critical shortage of nurses. And nurses can continue to practice nursing in new and exciting ways that allow their knowledge, experience, and skills from many years of professional work to be applied in different and potentially more efficient ways to provide patient care. The vision of this book is that of a growing cadre of vital senior nurses continuing to develop personally and professionally, addressing the growing needs of the expanding society and ranks of seniors, and improving the quality of health care.

This book is meant to be a resource for nurses and hospital administrators as well as an information source for the public. It is designed to highlight the value of older nurses and what they can offer the population as a resource for quality nursing care during this time of a critical shortage of nurses and in the future. It addresses the developmental strengths and needs of senior nurses, what they can offer during this most critical time, and ways they can determine their next career as a nurse. Unfortunately, for a variety of reasons, many nurses do not know what they want to do next, what skills they have that could contribute to their "next" career, and how they can learn about both.

We, the authors of this book, present a new and rapidly growing concept of the life course and activities of persons 50-75 years old, known by some as the Third Age. Our focus is on nurses who are reaching 50 years of age and need to plan for their future. Throughout the chapters are real-life stories that illustrate the lives and work of persons in the Third Age who have discovered ways to fulfill themselves while continuing to contribute to society's needs.

The book is organized as follows:

- In Chapter 1, we define the Third Age and describe six principles of growth and renewal in the Third Age. This chapter includes a practical application of these principles in Third Age Life Planning and building a Third Age Life/Work Portfolio.

- Chapter 2 explains how retirement has been changing in the United States and how the principles from Third Age Life Planning can aid nurses in redefining retirement and building a retirement transition.

- Chapters 3, 4, and 5 provide practical guidance for nurses interested in developing their careers in new ways.

- Chapter 6 explores how hospitals can develop strategies, policies, and practices to sustain and retain Third Age nurses.

- The book ends with Chapter 7, a chapter on how the nurses of today can create a nurse workforce for tomorrow that can have a major impact on health care and the kind of workplace that will employ these future nurses.

The major contribution of this book is to clearly demonstrate the value of Third Age nurses and the strategies they can use to change the course of their lives, their careers, and the health care delivery system.

References

Buerhaus, P. (2008). Current and future state of the US nursing workforce. *The Journal of the American Medical Association, 300*(20), 2422-2424.

Federwisch, A. (June 2, 2008). Holy Names center helps rejuvenate older nurses' careers. *NurseWeek*. Retrieved March 18, 2009 from http://include.nurse.com/apps/pbcs.dll/article?AID=/20080602/CA02/80529003

When Retirement Isn't The Answer

Growing Older in the 21ˢᵗ Century | 1

A New Paradigm of Aging

The shape and quality of human life after the age of 50 have changed dramatically during the past 100 years. In fact, we have been experiencing a *longevity revolution*. In the United States, life expectancy jumped from 47 years in 1900 to more than 77 years in 2000. That's a 30-year life "bonus" for the second half of life! And that number keeps going up. According to U.S. Census data, American life expectancy has increased to 78, and women turning 65 years old in 2007 had an average of 20 more years of life ahead of them. American men, whose life expectancy has trailed women on average by about 5 years, are beginning to catch up. The 2008 Central Intelligence Agency World Fact Book reports at least 11 countries today with an average life expectancy of over 80 years. A third of the citizens in some countries are over 65. Marc Freedman, author of the 2007 book *Encore: Finding Work That Matters in the Second Half of Life* and creator of the Web site Encore Careers, predicts that Americans turning 65 now will live to see their 90th birthday. In the United States and many other countries, the over-85 population is expanding rapidly. But the fastest growing population group in the United States now consists of centenarians. In 1965, there were just 3,000 centenarians; in 2000, the number ballooned to 70,000. According to the U.S. Census Bureau, the number of centenarians by 2050 will be 1.1 million, especially if 78 million baby boomers take charge of their lives to stay physically, mentally, and socially active and healthy.

Most people in the second half of life have more years ahead of them than anyone imagined just 30 years ago. This fact is an extremely important change in the life course; everyone over 50 should recognize and act upon this change, especially health care professionals. Everyone needs to build a longevity strategy, and the sooner a person builds a strategy for positive aging, the better, not only for personal but for social reasons. Some economists and demographic forecasters have pointed to dire social consequences with a greatly expanded population of seniors—greater longevity could squeeze the life out of the economy. If 78 million baby boomers live longer but age poorly, health care costs could break the federal budget.

But these dire forecasts are predicated on a pattern of aging that prevailed in the past and have not adequately considered a new paradigm. There is an alternative future for aging.

Scientific studies have confirmed diverse patterns in aging; in fact people age differently (Baltes & Baltes, 1990). Until recently, aging has been associated with illness and disparagingly defined with *D* words such as decline, degeneration, deterioration, dementia, disengagement, depression, disease, disability, and dependency (Sadler, 2000). In their book *Successful Aging*, John W. Rowe and Robert L. Kahn refer to this old, negative view of aging as "usual aging" (Rowe & Kahn, 1998). However, an entirely new paradigm of aging is becoming apparent, pointing to positive development after 60, 70, 80, and even 90. Even centenarians have demonstrated sustained healthy development rather than degeneration (Perls & Silver, 2000).

Recognizing a New View of Aging

Gerontological research has been destroying myths and assumptions about aging. Walter Bortz, a leader in vital aging, recommends that *we dare to be 100* (Bortz, 1996). The conventional image of an old person as frail, sickly, and sometimes demented has now been recognized as just one possibility that we should actively and thoughtfully avoid. The exciting news from both research and everyday observations of vital, healthy, active, productive older citizens is that an entirely new possibility of aging exists—if we actively take charge of our own life course. Various terms have been coined to name this new gerontological phenomenon of positive aging: *successful aging*, *creative aging*, *vital aging*, and *aging well*. The focus in this book is on the middle period of life stretching from 50 to 75, the *Third Age*.

Positive Aging Characteristics	Negative Aging Characteristics
Vibrant	Feeble
Healthy	Infirm
Wise	Demented
Competent	Disabled
Independent	Dependent
Creative	Rigid
Adventuresome	Timid
Engaged	Disengaged

How can we account for this emerging positive alternative? Some say longevity is in the genes, but genes alone cannot account for the rapid surge of longevity and healthy aging. Medical science and technology have certainly contributed. Research into successful aging has demonstrated the importance of thoughtful, disciplined health care; social engagement; meaningful activity; lifelong learning; and an infrastructure of strong interpersonal relationships and a social network. Life strategies

"Life strategies make a huge difference in how people experience the second half of life."

make a huge difference in how people experience the second half of life.

In addition, neuroscience has produced some startling discoveries about the "aging" brain in just the past 25 years. We previously believed the brain had a limited number of neurons, established at birth. Now we know the brain can produce both new neurons and new dendrites, the connecting synapses that support brain activity. Neuroscientists such as Michael Merzenich of Stanford University, and founder of a brain fitness company called PositScience, have shown the brain has unexpected plasticity to keep it operating vitally and effectively, which constitutes a cognitive basis for creative, productive, healthy development during the entire second half of life. Merzenich and his team of researchers argue that we need to keep our brains healthy and operating effectively by practicing *brain fitness* as well as physical fitness. (See http://www.positscience.com/science/studies_results/ for published and unpublished studies concerning brain functionality and aging.)

Psychiatrist Gene Cohen (2005), who has been studying the aging process for decades, maintains that people over 50 have an inner push toward healthy, creative growth, driven by what he calls *developmental intelligence*. In fact, the mature brain can continually re-sculpt itself with new cells, better circuitry, greater balance, and integration. But individuals need to commit themselves to sustaining their own cognitive development. If we seek and regularly respond to new challenges, we can sustain positive plasticity and full-fledged personal development; otherwise, we risk promoting the negative brain plasticity that we often see in usual aging. The discovery of positive neurodevelopment in people over 50 provides the mechanism to explain new options for development after 50; the mature brain establishes a basis for renewed youthfulness, expanding creativity and personal fulfillment.

The new paradigm of positive aging challenges long-held assumptions and expectations about what is in store for us after passing 50 or 60 or 70. What does *old* mean now? In the paradigm of usual aging, old age was said to begin at 60. But now, we see 60-year-olds developing new interests and skills; engaging in creative and productive work; staying fit and active; engaging in vigorous forms of work and play; acquiring a variety of knowledge and insights; and building new families, friendships, and communities. Some say 60 is the new 40 or 50. Or maybe it's just a new 60, one that is radically different from the old pattern. The good news about positive aging is of great importance to everyone, especially those in health care professions committed to the promotion of health and well-being. Aging just isn't what it used to be—*if we do it right.*

> "Some say 60 is the new 40 or 50. Or maybe it's just a new 60, one that is radically different from the old pattern."

Committing to a New View of Life After 50

In 25 years of research following people who have been changing course in the second half of their lives, Sadler has been discovering people who illustrate the new paradigm of positive aging in the Third Age. Rebecca, though not a nurse, provides an example of a person who has tapped her creative potential to redesign her life and her work to experience years of fulfillment (Sadler & Krefft, 2008). After she graduated from the University of Texas, Rebecca thought she would develop a career in university theatrical production. However, after a few years in this field, she met a European emigrant who wooed her and won her hand in marriage. They moved first to New England, where he finished a graduate degree, which led to work in an international company in San Francisco, California. When that company collapsed, he started his own company, and they began to build a family. Rebecca settled into a role of wife and mother, caring for three growing children.

After a dozen years, with the children all in school, her husband persuaded her to work for his mail-order company as merchandising manager. So at 38, she entered a new career as a manager in a for-profit company. Although she had no previous experience in this line of work, she found that many skills she had acquired in theatrical production also applied to merchandising. She threw herself into this work for the next 20 years, balancing her new career with family responsibilities. When she turned 58, Rebecca noted she had given her family and the family business her time, talents, and energy. "Now it's time for me," she said to herself and her husband. She was not interested in retiring—a term she and her husband disliked and avoided. What she wanted was the opportunity to develop her creative capacities and interests.

As a young mother, she had taken some art courses and had discovered she had the potential to become an artist. During her business career, she had put that possibility on hold. After leaving the company, she enrolled in an art institute, where she progressed rapidly in a variety of artistic media: painting, sculpting, sketching, and crafts. By age 76, nearly 20 years after "retiring" from her job, she had produced an impressive portfolio of artwork. Her works have been shown in galleries at San Francisco's city hall and public library and featured in community projects. Painting became her primary work in her 60s and 70s. Her *work* has been redefined as an expression of her passion and new personal identity.

As she was developing into a productive, recognized artist, she also learned an entirely new athletic skill—playing tennis. She started playing nearly every day, taking lessons and practicing to improve her performance on the court. In her 60s, she was captain of a team that won a national championship in the Super Senior Tennis League. At 77, she still plays tennis and exercises regularly by hiking the hills around San Francisco. With her husband, she also became involved in several charitable and philanthropic projects. Now that her children are grown and raising their own children, she devotes more time to being a grandmother. She prepares a weekly family meal where three generations gather for food, fun, and conversation. Rebecca models vital, creative, successful aging within her Third Age—she exemplifies all the positive traits we see in the new paradigm of positive aging. She has consciously developed a longevity strategy for a new period in the middle of life that is radically different from the old paradigm of usual aging.

In the course of writing this book we have encountered nurses who, like Rebecca, decided they wanted to change course in their 50s. Frank, for example, served as a full-time nurse in a large metropolitan hospital, eventually working his way up to a position as an executive nurse. He was challenged and satisfied by his professional work, but in his mid-50s, Frank began to sense it was time to explore other possibilities. He left his job and moved his family to rural New England, where he found work teaching in a community college. This was an exciting new venture, but after 3 years on a self-designed sabbatical, he was ready to return to nursing. However, he was not interested in nursing in the same way he did previously. He negotiated with the hospital administration a different kind of work relationship, with fewer hours, more flexibility, and a new focus. He now works 8-hour shifts 3 days a week and spends the fourth day at home doing research and grant writing. Several years ago he won a prestigious, large grant to design a special residency program for nurses, to build teams to learn about effective ways to provide geriatric nursing. He has shaped his work to suit the way he wants to live, and at 65 he is fully engaged in a long-term project to provide an innovative form of health care as well as a supportive learning program for nurse colleagues.

Helen illustrates a similar adventure in redesigning her life and work after 50. In addition to a full-time nursing career in suburban New Jersey, she was a wife and mother of two girls. As her girls were finishing high school, Helen returned to school to earn a degree that would qualify her for promotion to an administrative position. She took on a new role, but realized that she was inspired by graduate learning and research. So she enrolled in a doctoral program, where she honed her research skills. After completing her doctoral program, she found work in a large New York hospital, where she led a new program in evidence-based practice with a special focus on geriatric nursing. Like Frank, she has shaped an entirely new career, fulfilling her personal needs while at the same time providing leadership in an innovative approach in health care. Nurses such as Helen and Frank are experiencing new possibilities, opportunities, and challenges that are emerging in a new period in the middle of life, the *Third Age*.

What Does the Third Age Signify in the Changing Life Course?

As the average life course extends significantly with greater longevity and adds quality in the final decades with vital, successful aging, an entirely new period is emerging that replaces middle age and early usual aging. Some writers have said it is a season in life that seeks a purpose and needs a name. We believe that a useful name is the *Third Age*; its purpose is to afford us with the opportunity for personal growth, ongoing contributions, and fulfillment. It follows the *Second Age*, which focuses on achievement, and precedes the *Fourth Age*, which is for life completion.

Third Age is a widely used term in Europe, Australia, New Zealand, and Canada to designate the period of retirement. For many Third Age Life Coaches, it signifies much more. It represents a new opportunity and challenge for significant personal growth from 50 to 80. Before 50, life is largely shaped by compulsion; we are driven by what we have to do to survive and to achieve success. A healthy, meaningful Third Age is shaped by choices.

Sadler has spent 25 years investigating human development in the Third Age. He began his research shortly after entering his 50s, because he was puzzled by the discrepancy between what he was personally experiencing and seeing in the lives of some of his peers and what the literature on human development was describing and predicting. At that time, the life course was seen to follow an upward curve until about 50, followed by a decline—adult development up to 50, then aging in the usual sense. He set out to learn if there might be an alternative model for adult life, one where development did not stop but in fact continued. And if it continued, how did it continue? He began to interview people in their late 40s and early 50s who seemed to be thriving, not declining, as they moved into the second half of life. After interviewing about 200 people, he focused on several dozen who seemed to be setting a new example of vital, creative, purposeful living. They were growing impressively and breaking the old model. The direction of their lives was up, not down. Most had reached a peak earlier in their lives and were now aiming for new peaks. He tracked these people for a dozen years, asking, "What are they doing to initiate and sustain this unexpected growth?" After analysis, both quantitative and qualitative, he concluded that they had a handful of qualities in common. These qualities, the six principles of second growth, form the central message of his 2000 book, *The Third Age: Six Principles of Growth and Renewal After 40.*

- Principle 1: Mindful reflection and risk-taking

- Principle 2: Realistic optimism

- Principle 3: Building a positive Third Age identity

■ Principle 4: Redefining and balancing work and play

■ Principle 5: Expanding and balancing personal freedom and intimacy

■ Principle 6: Building a more caring life with caring for others, for self, for the world

From the people he studied, whose stories fill the book and illustrate the principles, he learned important lessons about alternatives to usual patterns of middle age and aging. Perhaps the most important challenge for those in the Third Age is learning to tap their creative potential to sustain second growth, allowing them to experience fulfillment and make a difference in the world. The old models of middle aging and usual aging are not normal; they represent just one possibility. We have a choice to go a different route. By creatively designing our lives in the Third Age and following these principles, we can also build a foundation for positive, successful aging in the Fourth Age.

> "The old models of middle aging and usual aging are not normal; they represent just one possibility. We have a choice to go a different route."

The Six Principles in Third Age Growth

What Sadler has called second growth in the Third Age differs from personal growth in the first half of life. Instead of moving step by step in a linear pattern from stage to stage, second growth spirals around key issues, often moving in apparently contradictory or paradoxical directions. The principles, which are responses to the key issues, can be used to help launch and sustain one's growth. How they operate can be most easily understood by following just one person, Ted, whose life over the past 20 years so clearly illustrates all of the principles (Sadler, 2000; Sadler & Krefft, 2008). His unfolding life, both professional and personal, has many elements that nurses can identify with and learn from. Before deciding on a life direction after 50, nurses should set decisions about work and retirement within a larger context of Third Age Life Planning based on the six principles. There is no one right way to apply the principles, nor do the principles necessarily follow in order from one through six. But, the first two principles provide a foundation that can be applied in any person's life to four key areas in the last four principles.

Principle 1: Mindful Reflection and Risk-Taking

As he approached 50, Ted had been an architect for nearly 25 years, working with a growing firm founded by one of his graduate school professors. His first marriage, which produced three children, lasted just 12 years, in part because he was overly committed to his career. He subsequently married a woman who shared his professional and artistic interests, but after 10 years, this marriage also began to show problems. At this time, Ted went on an Outward Bound wilderness course, where a probing self-examination led him to realize his life was "out of whack." He had no balance; he often put in 100-hour weeks, even working on major holidays. He began asking the kinds of questions that lead to positive growth: *Where am I going? What do I want? What are my core values? What's most important? What have I been leaving out? What do I need to do next?* These questions formed the basis for ongoing mindful reflection about the meaning, purpose, and shape of the next phase in his life.

By the end of the course, Ted came up with his own life design. He used the metaphor of a four-legged stool. The first leg was work. At that time, all the weight was on just this leg. The second leg was his marriage and family. The third leg was community service. The fourth leg was his health, well-being, and enjoyment. After reflection, he sketched out a plan. Then he had to make choices and take risks to initiate new behaviors. There is a paradox here, of quietly turning inward and then actively moving outward to make changes. Five years later, his life was balanced among all four values. The irony, he said, was that although he gave much more time to his family, the community, and his own well-being, the quality of his work actually improved.

Principle 2: Realistic Optimism

> "Virtually every study of healthy development and positive aging has affirmed the importance of having a confident, hopeful attitude toward life and one's self."

Virtually every study of healthy development and positive aging has affirmed the importance of having a confident, hopeful attitude toward life and one's self. But this attitude should be realistic, not a fantasy. Ted was brave enough to admit his life was moving in a direction that would founder if he did not make some radical changes. He acknowledged failures and the shadow side in his life, as well as the risks he would need to take in his career to achieve his dreams for a fulfilling marriage; a healthy lifestyle with more time for fun, creativity, and friendship; and greater involvement in important causes and deserving community projects. As he began to branch out in other areas of his life, he worked on improving his sense of confidence and hopefulness. Optimism was a driving force in his creative development.

Principle 3: Building a Positive Third Age Identity

Like many people in their Second Age, Ted had been focusing on achieving success, measured by external signs such as recognition, income, and status. Our personal identities as adults are shaped by the roles we play and our achievements within the roles. A burning question in the Second Age has been, "What do we want to do?" As we move into the second half of life, researchers such as Cohen and Sadler find people asking another question: "Who do I want to become?" Even successful, established people in their 50s and 60s sometimes have said, "I'm not sure who I want to be when I grow up." They are aware that the identity they have achieved in their Second Age needs revision for a fulfilling Third Age.

After 50, we find questions of meaning and purpose come to the forefront. In re-examining his life and career, Ted realized he had basically defined himself as an architect and as a partner in the firm. As the firm grew in size, the founder decided to simplify the firm's name by using just his own name, thereby removing the names of Ted and the other partners. In responding to what he first saw as a loss, Ted realized he wanted to define himself differently. Instead of seeing himself primarily as an architect and partner in the firm, he asked, "How can I achieve balance and become a whole person?" Like others who exhibit Third Age growth, he reinvented himself in the second half of life, shaping his growth around a set of core values and a sense of purpose. Forging a new personal identity, especially as a professional, requires redefining success. For Ted, this meant measuring success in terms of self-expression, relationships, meaning, learning, and contribution, not in terms of number of projects, accomplishments, income, and recognition. Ted redefined success as realizing his own fulfillment, rather than achieving external goals.

Another important element in redefining oneself consists of examining one's sense of age. As the famous African-American pitcher Satchel Paige quipped: "How old would you be if you didn't know how old you was?" As we pass 50, we are vulnerable to many negative cultural stereotypes about growing older. We don't live in a society that values older people; on the contrary, our culture has a fixation on youth. Being older does not yet resonate with value added. In the self-examination process, we need to explore the negative images of aging we have acquired. These old scripts interfere with our intention to keep growing; we should shred them and create new scripts for our unfolding lives. Ted was aware that he seemed much younger than his parents were at his age. He chose a different self-image for himself than they had for themselves at his age. At one point, he commented that his parents had apparently given in to the culturally defined sense of old age and were pulled down by it. He, however, sensed youthfulness within himself, a spirit that had been squeezed out of an over-committed professional career.

Part of his life design included more free time and play, so he could reaffirm a youthful spirit. He and his wife pursued common interests—painting, sailing, skiing, building a second home, entertaining friends, and spending time with his children and grandchildren. He also began taking better care of himself; at 65 he said he felt in better shape, stronger, and younger than he felt at 50. He accepted his aging, but at the same time he lived the paradox of growing younger as he grew older.

Principle 4: Redefining and Balancing Work and Play

One of the most significant surprises that researchers of this new period in life have encountered is the discovery that Third Age people have a different attitude toward work than we might have expected just 20 years ago. Instead of saying they want to quit work to retire, more people are saying work is becoming more important to them. But, it is work they have redefined to suit the way they choose to live, not some endeavor imposed and defined by someone else. Many recent studies of people facing retirement have made a similar discovery. People, especially baby boomers, have said they want to continue working in some capacity, pointing toward an entirely different conception of retirement.

Ted loved his work as an architect. It was a vehicle for creative expression and growth, a way to contribute to families and society, and a challenge to continue learning and mentoring, as well as a way to earn a living. In his Second Age, his career was consuming him, but in his Third Age, it became one important part of himself that was balanced with other values, interests, and commitments.

In crafting a new design in his work life, he deliberately set much more time for play. Because he was a former athlete, some of his play time involved sports. He regularly allowed time for golf and tennis with male friends, boating and skiing with his wife, and leisure activities with his children and grandchildren. But he also developed another form of play in sketching and painting. As he grew older, he also allowed more time for reading and conversation with family and friends.

Asked at age 60 if he had any plans to retire, he said, "No." Why should he stop what he loved doing? Also, he needed to continue earning an income. At 65, when he saw some of his peers retire, he began to reconsider. What was he to do next? He wanted more free time to pursue other interests, but he did not want to give up his practice altogether. So he negotiated a special contract with his firm to work 3 days in the middle of the week, leaving 4 days to spend with his wife, family, and friends and on special community projects. He became passionately concerned about the environment and conservation and worked with several organizations whose mission was to support and improve the environment, both in the wilderness and in cities. In addition to contributing his skills and talents to architectural projects and environmental causes, he also added a new career as a part-time teacher of landscape design at universities, and he became a mentor to younger architects, both in his firm and in internships. At 72, he saw no reason to stop doing what he loved; in fact, his redesigned career *felt like a promotion*. This is also what the new 70 looks like.

Principle 5: Expanding and Balancing Personal Freedom and Intimacy

Over and over researchers have heard people say that after 50, they value a greater sense of personal freedom more than ever. Similar to Sadler, Cohen has also found that a first phase in development after 50 is an experience of liberation. Ted, for example, wanted more freedom *from* his fixation on a career. In addition to freedom from, he wanted more freedom *to*—to move in new directions, attend to a variety of interests, explore other avenues, and become more inventive and experimental. This liberation is not a midlife crisis, but an existential, even spiritual movement toward meaning and purpose. As with others, Ted's increased freedom was also a way to experience greater intimacy with his wife, children, friends, and colleagues. Enlarging *freedom to* enables one's life to be shaped by choice rather than by necessity and compulsion. With more freedom, Ted was able to build a much closer relationship with his wife. At 55 he reported they had a perfect marriage; he said the same at 70. When he was all wrapped up in his career, he had experienced alienation from his children. With more freedom, he renewed his relationships with his children; as they matured, married, and produced children, he was intimately involved in their lives and has developed close relationships with eight grandchildren. And like others in studies of positive aging, he has formed and sustained close friendships.

Principle 6: Building a More Caring Life With Caring for Others, for Self, for the World

George Vaillant, a psychiatrist and author of a leading study of aging well, has found in longitudinal studies of three very different populations that a key ingredient in positive aging is *generativity* (Vaillant, 2002). This term, originally coined by psychologist Erik Erikson, refers to a distinctive personality trait appearing in people over 50; it means caring for those who are coming after or the younger generation. As Vaillant and others apply the term, its scope is much broader—children, parents, families, colleagues, the socially disadvantaged, the world, and the future.

Ted's story reflects an impressive development of generativity in his family, his workplace, and the community. The growth of generative caring grows out of deep, personal questions: *What and who do I really care about? What legacy am I going to leave?* His work with environmental groups expressed his concern for the future of our planet. He altered the focus of his job, adding a significant portion of time to mentor young architects. He also became more involved in the lives of his grandchildren.

Ted's developing life also expresses another paradox. As he expanded caring for others, the world, and this planet, he also devoted more time and energy to caring for himself. He set up a regimen to establish a healthy lifestyle in his 50s. He had been eating too much and drinking too much alcohol, so he cut down on both. He also began to exercise regularly, not only in sports but also at a fitness center. He began to take daily walks of several miles, often with his wife. In his 60s, he had a hip replacement; his doctor advised him to take off more weight. He lost 30 pounds, which made him feel better, stronger, and more youthful. At 70 he was as active as he had been in his 50s; the only exceptions were that he cut out horseback riding and black diamond downhill ski runs.

Edward Schneider, a member of the MacArthur Foundation Study of Successful Aging and former dean of the Leonard Davis School of Gerontology at the University of Southern California, has identified six important areas to address to sustain vital, healthy, positive aging (Schneider & Miles, 2003):

- Nutrition
- Exercise
- Weight
- Sleep
- Social engagement
- Hormones

Nurses and Third Age

The potential for Third Age growth to be a foundation for positive aging has inspired many people. While authors can stimulate minds to think about changing course, the actual change needs disciplined responses to the challenges. Transforming oneself is hard work, and most of us need some help. Many people have received help in creating a new direction from counselors, mentors, role models, therapists, and personal coaches, as well as wise friends and spouses. Nurses are doubly positioned to play an instrumental role in Third Age planning, both from a personal/professional standpoint and from their influence on health care consumers. Nursing is a physically, emotionally, and personally demanding career. Burn-out rates for nurses attest to that. Not only can nurses help others successfully transition to Third Age growth, but every nurse can benefit from this reflective and forward planning. With the average age of nurses in the United States over 46 years of age and 41% of the nursing population 50 or older, (United States Department of Health and Human Services, 2007), everyone in nursing has a vested interest in ensuring that qualified and talented nurses are not lost to traditional retirement, but can instead be redirected to other rewarding jobs and careers in nursing.

> "Transforming oneself is hard work, and most of us need some help."

Holy Names University's Center for Third Age Nurses has identified the critical considerations for nurses 50 and older as:

- Most nurses at this stage in their careers still love nursing.

- They do not love their specific jobs; they often are feeling burned out.

- They want to contribute to the health care profession, but they want to do something different now. They also are not in a position to leave work because they need the income.

- They do not know where to go to learn about and plan for other options.

Third Age Life Planning

Shortly after publication of *The Third Age: Six Principles of Growth and Renewal After 40*, a group of business professionals started a new enterprise to apply the six principles to the workforce. The Center for Third Age Leadership (www.ThirdAgeCenter.com) offers workshops, seminars, and retreats to individuals to help them get started. When the center's leaders realized that people aspiring to second growth need a long-term strategy, they added personal life coaches. These coaches design ongoing programs to assist individuals with practical application of the key ideas and principles of second growth. There is also an independent network of Third Age Life Coaches around the world; the appendix provides contact information for some of its leaders.

What has emerged is a new process, called *Third Age Life Planning,* which guides people in their second growth. An international network of coaches now specializes in this kind of planning. Workshops available through the Center for Third Age Nurses at Holy Names University introduce life planning to senior nurses who are asking questions about the post-50 phase in their lives. Five tasks are related to this planning (Sadler & Krefft, 2008).

- Task 1: Do your homework.

- Task 2: Change your negative images of aging.

- Task 3: Redefine success.

- Task 4: Build a new Third Age identity.

- Task 5: Create a Third Age infrastructure.

Task 1: Do Your Homework

The first step in life planning for second growth is to ask a lot of questions. *Where do I want to go with my life? What are my core values, interests, and aspirations? What talents and resources do I have to enable me to move in the desired direction?* To make dreams a reality, people also need to make realistic assessments about their investments, pension plans, health plans, and organizational policies that will affect income and employment. Guides to life planning are critically important, but with a rapidly changing economic situation, most people also need help with financial planning. Baby boomers especially have been noted to under-plan and under-invest for a long retirement. Many people have wrongly assumed they will have enough income to support a desired lifestyle; they haven't done their homework.

Good financial planners can help people realistically assess their needs and resources and design a strategy that can keep them solvent as they move toward or enter retirement. What nurses might not know is that recently, some significant changes in pre-retirement policies have occurred that can support their change of course (Byham, 2007). Until now, most organizations had an all or nothing policy—either you worked full time at your job or you left to take retirement or work elsewhere. More and more organizations have changed their employment options to allow greater flexibility. Increasingly, individuals can redesign their work to better suit the way they choose to live. In their 50s and 60s, many people, including senior nurses, want to downshift their work life; they want to work fewer hours with greater flexibility. In doing so, their income decreases. They then must find a way to have enough money to sustain their lifestyle and care for their families. Some pension funds now allow people to draw from their accounts before retirement, so that even with a reduced earned income, they can pay the bills. *Doing your homework* means getting reliable, up-to-date information about your health, income, insurance, pension, and employment options.

Task 2: Change Your Negative Images of Aging

Interviews and Third Age retreats have revealed that most people carry negative images of what it will be like to grow older. In spite of the news about positive development after 50, stereotypes of aging abound in our culture. Birthday cards reflecting a gallows humor about aging are plentiful in the so-called humorous card sections. Pharmaceutical companies exploit negative views and fears with daily ads in the media. Growing up in our culture has taught us many wrong lessons about aging. Everyday experience shows many people whose aging follows the "d" words—decline, disability, degeneration, deterioration, dementia, disengagement, depression, disease, and dependency—in the diminishing pattern of aging. That has been the pattern of usual aging, and nurses see many examples of such aging, but alternatives do exist. To move forward in a healthy, spirited way, we need to dispel old scripts—old beliefs—that can hold us back.

People who have followed a course of second growth show how they have battled these images. As we saw in Ted's case, he reflected on how his parents had succumbed to their assumptions about an enfeebled old age; he consciously chose to promote a more youthful way to grow older. He played more, kept himself physically fit, and planned regular "fun" activities with his wife, friends, and grandchildren. Like so many others in the examples of second growth, he looked forward to new adventures.

Susan is especially articulate about battling negative stereotypes. A single woman, Susan had achieved a career peak in her 50s by becoming a bank vice president for human resources, but when the bank merged with another, she was forced to leave. She was also diagnosed with cancer and underwent a complete hysterectomy. This double loss was a significant setback. But, she had always been optimistic and resilient, so she developed a plan to sustain her health and growth. She decided to join a pilgrimage in Greece to visit sites of ancient goddess civilizations. While on this pilgrimage, she said she was "relearning who I am, being born again through my discovery and embracing both the power and vulnerability of the feminine within me" (Sadler & Krefft, 2008, p. 195). When she returned, she decided to establish her own consulting company for organizational renewal and integrate her core feminine principles into her work with companies. She strove to provide leadership and leadership development programs that were consistent with her core values.

When she turned 60, the conventional beginning of old age, she was still developing a new sense of self. Susan resented the negative image of aging in our culture and was determined to sustain a healthy, vibrant lifestyle. She switched to a mostly vegetarian diet and began an exercise routine that included daily walks of several miles, yoga and fitness center workouts once or twice a week, and bike riding and kayaking when weather permitted. Along with physical fitness, she practiced brain fitness. At 65 she enrolled in a PhD program and completed her doctorate when she reached 70. In one interview, she made an eloquent statement about how she felt about her age:

> I resent the negative stereotypes of aging in our culture. I don't think of myself as old or feeble or diminished. There are many things I want to do, explore, and give before I die. I hope I have time to do it all. I feel some aches and pains and know I have to work with them and take care of them lovingly. I get up each day with a sense of gratitude and hope. I work on staying strong and healthy, because I want to be able to move the watering hose and carry my groceries into my nineties (Sadler & Krefft, 2008, p. 201).

Resisting the negative images of aging and affirming her renewed sense of self, Susan looked forward to living and aging well into her 90s. As a caring, engaged professional who has balanced ongoing service with personal fulfillment, and who consciously battles negative stereotypes of aging to build a positive Third Age identity, Susan could be a role model for nurses seeking to do something similar.

Task 3: Redefine Success

For most of our lives, we have measured success with the conventional icons of achievement, influence, and income and with a plethora of status symbols. The markers of success have been extrinsic. In the second half of life, the markers become intrinsic. A challenge in the Third Age is to redefine success in terms of fulfillment. That is easier said than done. After leaving a successful position or career, people often feel lost. As one recently retired senior manager of a large corporation quipped, "How are you supposed to transition from being somebody to being a nobody?" Recent studies of people approaching or entering retirement have found that a major issue at this time of life becomes developing a sense of purpose and meaning (Bratter & Dennis, 2008). The way ahead involves more probing questions about values, what really matters, and long-term aspirations.

"A challenge in the Third Age is to redefine success in terms of fulfillment."

El, a corporate financial manager approaching his 50th birthday, decided he needed to change course, because his 26-year career with the company was not allowing him to develop his creative potential. In a wellness seminar, he focused on the purpose of his life and came up with this statement: "The purpose of my life is to become the person I can be, to develop my potential and to share" (Sadler, 2000, p. 60). That realization led him to plan with his wife an entirely different life, away from Boston and in the place they had long dreamed about, a farm in Maine. During the next 20 years, they built a small antique business and blueberry farm, contributed to their community through volunteer work, started creative enterprises to develop young leaders and promote conservation, and helped develop a center to provide a living legacy of civic and environmental values. Success for El came to mean finding new opportunities and challenges to develop his potential and make meaningful contributions. "Success happens every day when I wake up and realize I have the ability to do whatever I choose and have lots of great things to choose from," he said. About 20 years after the initial interview, El summed up his successful transition into a new way of life this way:

> After leaving the company, I had not yet realized how much growth and renewal there was in store for us. I have so much enjoyed the chance to share my love of the outdoors, especially with youngsters, to leave our environment in a better state than I found it, to share the history and traditions of this region with future generations, to love my family more deeply, and to leave a legacy in this region of greater understanding and valuing of our rich outdoor heritage (Sadler & Krefft, 2008, p. 102).

In redefining success, these Third Age pioneers have designed a very individual pursuit of happiness. Questions asked of them were as follows: *What makes your soul sing? That is, what is your passion? How do you express it? Where do you feel exhilaration, joy, and fulfillment?* These emotions are intrinsic markers of success. In more than a quarter of a century studying happiness, psychologist Mihaly Csikszentmihalyi has described an optimal experience he calls *flow*. In moments of flow, people are engaged in a challenging activity that is neither too easy nor too difficult, where they become completely absorbed by what they are doing. In flow, people test their talents and skills, realize their potential, and experience happiness. People such as Susan, El, and Ted have redefined success to give themselves a maximum amount of flow in their lives. They engage often in activities that make their souls sing.

Task 4: Build a New Third Age Identity

When you are transitioning into the second half of life, the core principle in Third Age growth and renewal is forming a new personal identity. As we have seen, this involves seeing yourself not primarily in terms of roles and positions, but in terms of a renewing process to become the person you can be. Forming a new personal identity includes redefining success, replacing negative images of aging with a youthful sense of self that is integrated with growing older, and putting more flow into your life. A practical way of building a complex new identity is to see the process in terms of a Third Age Life Portfolio (Sadler & Krefft, 2008). You are the artist of your life, and with creative design you can assemble a complex balance of multiple interests and commitments that sustain second growth.

This book is primarily aimed at helping nurses rethink the course of their lives and redesign their work after 50. Until now the vast majority of books about this time in life have focused on financial planning, retirement planning, and/or new ways to work. But a new form of work should be set within the larger framework of Third Age planning that takes into consideration the key issues in a new paradigm of the Third Age and positive aging. A key concept in the life portfolio is a different model of working in the Third Age, what Sadler and Krefft (2008) have called Third Age Careers.

Underlying probing questions about what we want to do next in terms of work is a more fundamental question of meaning, values, and purpose: *Who do we want to become?* People such as Rebecca, Susan, El, and Ted have found fulfillment in their work and in their lives because they have creatively expanded their personal boundaries and effectively organized the paradoxical complexity of their mature personalities.

Third Age Life Portfolio

Third Age Life Coaches have set forth a practical framework for building such a portfolio.

1. Clarify your most important values and consider those moments in which you experience flow.

2. Identify those activities that express your core values and needs, challenge your talents, and support your growth.

3. Redirect your energies toward realizing your vision of who you want to become.

4. Apply this vision to your whole life, relating it to core areas found in the following list:

    - Significant relationships—spouse, family, best friends, neighbors, colleagues, clients, students, etc.

    - Self—core interests and talents, dreams and plans, learning, spirituality, and health.

    - Community service, helping others, and political action.

    - New forms of work—redefined as Third Age Careers—and ways to play, to laugh, and to be creative.

    - Location—home, travel, nature.

    - Favorite leisure activities.

Identifying key areas in your life that are currently important and those that you want to explore and expand can help you form a practical plan for growth and a design for a fulfilling Third Age.

Task 5: Create a Third Age Infrastructure

Redesigning your life for Third Age fulfillment is hard work, even harder than you might imagine. Because we grew up under the old model of usual aging, most of us are not prepared for our Third Age.

Those who engage in second growth in the Third Age are pioneers on a new frontier. Role models are scarce. The way ahead is untested. As people set a new course after 50, they need lots of support, reassurance, assistance, and feedback. One of the lessons learned from research is that we should not plan to travel the road ahead alone. We need to build an infrastructure, a social network that supports this new venture. As a single woman, Susan did not have a spouse to confide in, but she had a circle of close friends and a life coach with whom she could explore new ideas about her development. Ted and El had very supportive spouses; their married lives included regular time periods to share dreams, hopes, fears, and to explore ways they could keep building their life portfolios. Many people have engaged counselors, therapists, and financial planners to help them clarify intentions and make wise choices.

In addition to getting help from selected individuals, people need organizational support for their creative efforts to explore new pathways. Ted negotiated a different model of employment with his firm, so that he could continue to take on projects but have greater flexibility. Nurses also need to work with their employers to design different employment terms, so they can continue working in ways that are part of their own, unique Third Age Life Portfolio. Some people on the verge of retirement have negotiated a different employment relationship when the organization did not want to lose them. For example, a CEO told an insurance leader that he was too valuable to lose; together they designed a way for the leader to take on a completely different role to serve the company, with a much more flexible schedule (Sadler & Krefft, 2008).

Another way to build infrastructure is to become engaged in an organization that is specifically designed to help people change course. In response to a severe shortage of nurses in California, a group of nurse leaders took the initiative to form The Center for Third Age Nurses at

Holy Names University in Oakland, California. Their aim has been to help other senior nurses consider remaining in the health care system, rather than taking early retirement. The Center for Third Age Nurses has set out to inform senior nurses of options for new directions in work, to provide support for transition and personal transformation, and to build supportive networks between individual nurses and health care organizations to make needed changes. They have been engaged in a two-year planning operation to gather information, conduct focused interviews with senior nurses contemplating retirement, share findings within nursing organizations, and design interactive workshops to launch Third Age Life Planning for interested nurses.

Final Words

This chapter has argued that nurses should become aware of how the life course has changed in the 21st century, adding a new middle period from about 50 to 75 called the Third Age. As nurses reflect on what might develop in their lives as they think about careers, aging, and retirement, they should see a new era filled with possibilities, opportunities, and challenges. If people see what's possible after 50 and take responsibility for setting new directions, they can experience an era of great fulfillment. Based on the experience of Third Age pioneers, it is a good idea for nurses to engage in Third Age Life Planning. This involves applying the Six Principles of Growth and Renewal and the five steps just described. These set a positive framework for nurses to think about and design their own futures. Many nurses, as they pass 50, will find this framework helpful as they consider extending their professional careers beyond retirement age. In the process, nurses will also have to reconsider retirement, how it has been changing, and how they might redefine it for themselves.

References

Baltes, P., & Baltes, M. (Eds.) (1990). *Successful aging: Perspectives from the behavioral sciences*. Cambridge: Cambridge University Press.

Bortz, W. M. (1996). *Dare to be 100*. New York: Simon & Schuster.

Bratter, B., & Dennis, H. (2008). *Project renewment: The first retirement model for career women*. New York: Scribner.

Byham, W. C. (2007). *70—The new 50: Retirement management*. Pittsburgh, PA: DDI Press.

Centers for Disease Control and Prevention and The Merck Company Foundation. (2007). *The State of Aging and Health in America*. Whitehouse Station, NJ: The Merck Company Foundation; 2007.

Cohen, G. D. (2005). *The mature mind: The positive power of the aging brain*. New York: Basic Books.

Csikszentmihalyi, M. (1990). *Flow: The psychology of optimal experience*. New York: Harper & Rowe.

Freedman, M. (2007). *Encore: Finding work that matters in the second half of life*. New York: Public Affairs.

Mahncke, H.W., Bronstone, A., & Merzenich, M.M. (2006). Brain plasticity and functional losses in the aged: Scientific bases for a novel intervention. *Progress in Brain Research*. 2006; 157:81-109.

Merzenich, Michael. (2007). www.PositScience.com.

Perls, T., & Silver, M. (2000). *Living to 100: Lessons in living to your maximum potential at any age*. New York: Basic Books.

Rowe, J., & Kahn, R. (1998). *Successful aging*. New York: Pantheon.

Sadler, W. A. (2000). *The Third Age: Six principles of growth and renewal after 40*. Cambridge, MA: Perseus Books.

Sadler, W. A., & Krefft, J. H. (2008). *Changing course: Navigating life after 50*. Centennial, CO: The Center for Third Age Leadership Press.

Schneider, E., & Miles, E. (2003). *Ageless: Take control of your age and stay youthful for life*. New York: Rodale.

United States Census Bureau. (2009). The American FactFinder. Retrieved January 29, 2009 from http://factfinder.census.gov/home/saff/main.html?_lang=en

United States Department of Health and Human Services. (2007). *The registered nurse population: Findings from the 2004 national sample survey of registered nurses.* Retrieved January 6, 2009, from http://bhpr.hrsa.gov/health-workforce/rnsurvey04/

Vaillant, G. (2002). *Aging well: Surprising guideposts to a happier life from the landmark Harvard study of adult development.* Boston: Little-Brown.

Rethinking Retirement for Nurses | 2

As millions of older Americans approach retirement, many ponder the possibility of finding a safe, secure mooring within it. However, others wonder whether retirement is what they really want. They are asking searching questions that are not readily answered. *What's next in life for me? Is retirement really where I want to go? If so, can I afford it? What does it offer me? Where might it lead? What might I lose if I choose to take it when it's available? What other options do I have?*

The Changing View of Retirement

More and more people, especially nurses, are beginning to think that retirement is not the direction they want to take at this point in their lives. Interviews with senior nurses have shown that most are unsure of what retirement might mean for them. Many are ambivalent. If they retire, they might get relief from some undesirable parts of their jobs, but they will also lose aspects they value, such as providing a service, camaraderie, opportunities for learning, a sense of purpose, and, of course, their income. A common concern many have is what they will do with their time. Especially with an economic recession, most express concern about finances in a retirement that could last much longer than had previously been planned for. Will they have enough retirement income to sustain a desired lifestyle?

Many people have concluded that retirement, as we have known it, is not a good idea—at least not for them. Twenty years ago, in their last book that was promoting a more dynamic view of aging, Erik and Joan Erikson noted that retirement "seems to doom a large segment of our population to inertia and inactivation" (Erikson & Erikson, 1986, p. 297). The term itself does not suggest anything positive. It comes from a French word that means withdrawal; it suggests a condition similar to an old, worn-out book that has been pulled from circulation and stored on a back shelf. Sadler and Krefft found that all the subjects they followed in their research had a negative view of retirement (2008). Like those individuals they describe in their book, many people are already pursuing a different course, one that offers opportunities for new forms of work and challenges for self-discovery and growth.

How Has Retirement Evolved in the United States?

Retirement is a fairly new institution that increased exponentially during the 20th century. Before that a few men, perhaps elder statesmen, retired from their professions to enter a life of leisure because they could afford to, but nearly everyone else had to keep working. In 1900, most men 65 years old or older were still in the workforce; they had to remain employed to survive. Older women, if not enfeebled or sick, also worked in jobs and in their homes until the end of their days. But during the Great Depression, a third of the nation could not find steady employment. To be old at that time often meant to live in poverty. When President Franklin D. Roosevelt signed the Social Security Act in 1935, he sought to provide an income to people age 65 and older, who could then retire from the workforce. Retirees would get a well-deserved rest from labor, and employment opportunities would increase for young workers.

Our modern American version of retirement as a nearly universal phenomenon for older workers began after World War II. By 1950, most men who had reached 65 had started taking Social Security payments; just 46% remained in the workforce. Most of the women who had flooded into the workforce during the war had returned to their homes. During the 1950s and 1960s, more people found retirement to be an option because it was finally affordable. In many cases, retirement was mandatory upon reaching 65. New policies forced people of retirement age to leave their jobs and professions, whether they wanted to or not. So how did they support themselves? In addition to Social Security benefits, many people had retirement funds with defined benefits that gave them a guaranteed, albeit modest, income. In addition, some people had savings to draw from. These combined resources enabled older citizens to live comfortably, or at least stay out of poverty, without working. So, relatively new financial resources allowed a large majority of people to retire in their 60s. In the 1980s, the average retirement age declined dramatically to 62, in contrast to age 74 in 1910 (Giandrea, Cahill, & Quinn, 2007). By 1990, men older than 65 constituted a mere 3% of the workforce. Just 15% of them continued to work, and a third of these men worked only part time.

A Life Without Work

During the second half of the 20th century, retirement for people older than 55 came to be understood as a single event that led to a life *without work;* retirement basically meant *not working.* Gradually it acquired an additional, more glamorous meaning. As people began to live longer, healthier lives, a cultural shift began to redefine retirement along more attractive lines. A leader in this movement was Del Webb, a dynamic real estate investor who created and developed Sun City, Arizona, which promoted a life of leisure for seniors who had finished their working days. Webb constructed sprawling housing projects exclusively for seniors, who were retiring with pensions, savings, and Social Security. He named this new style of retirement the *Golden Years*. His definition reached far beyond the special communities he built. Retirement gradually came to mean a life dedicated to leisure (Freedman, 1999). The millions of people who flooded into his and other retirement communities around the country were provided with entertainment and structured activities to fill their leisured lives. Although only 5% of seniors actually moved into retirement communities such as those designed by Webb, his vision was widely adopted and became an inspiration for an aging generation—so much so that during the 1970s and 1980s, more people sought to take early retirement, before reaching 65. By the end of the century, retirement was a huge institution that absorbed nearly everyone 65 and over, with more and more people in their early 60s joining their ranks. The Golden Years had become an aspirational model for the nation.

"A serious challenge for retired people has been what to do with all the time on their hands."

But most Americans are not prepared for a life of leisure. A serious challenge for retired people has been what to do with all the time on their hands. Observers of communities such as Sun City have commented on what they perceived to be an almost frenetic busyness of residents, who were packing their days with scheduled activities provided by management. However, many citizens experienced empty days and curtailed lives. A 1997 Penn State University study of seniors found that most spent their abundance of free time watching television and gardening (Freedman, 2007). Other observers have noted that many retirees seem to have made a new career of golf. Surveys have reported that some retirees admit feeling marginal, useless, and adrift, not knowing what to do with themselves. Being retired has been described as a "role-less role," leaving people with nothing significant to do and a decimated personal identity. In spite of the glamour Del Webb attributed to a leisured life in the Golden Years, many retirees have experienced a deficit of meaning and a withering sense of purpose. The ideal that Webb created—which still is promoted widely in the media and by financial institutions—has become tarnished. In 1997, even a Sun City survey reported many retirees were longing for a life that offered more than just endless weekends (Freedman, 1999 and 2007). Thus, we do not find it surprising that many people approaching retirement age, including senior nurses, are having second thoughts about this phase in their lives.

A Different Kind of Retirement

As life expectancy increased dramatically in the latter part of the 20th century, the modern American version of elderly leisure could no longer be sustained. Marc Freedman, author and promoter of a radically different view of retirement, observed that leisure cannot support a long period in the middle of life. The early notion of a "well-deserved rest from labor" and the later notion of years spent busily pursuing fun in senior compounds come up short. Freedman's Civic Ventures (www.civicventures.org) survey of a thousand Americans between the ages of 50 and 70 found an emerging alternative aspiration—a widespread desire for meaningful work to create a better world. His institute has recognized and promoted new kinds of careers, careers in which people can find work that matters by making significant social contributions, often on a volunteer basis. Freedman has argued that the conventional notion of retirement needs to be replaced with a re-designed life with new forms of work that provide meaning and allow people to leave a legacy. A life consumed by leisurely fun or abundant inactivity does not meet people's deepest needs.

During the 1990s, a counterculture critical of the conventional notion of retirement began to emerge. More older people have sought to create alternatives to the Golden Years. Some have invented new names for retirement to go with different lifestyles, such as *refirement*, *protirement*, and *graduation* (Sadler & Krefft, 2008). Those inventing these new terms have sought a word that suggests moving on with passion, going forward in a positive direction, and successfully completing a career to commence a new course with great opportunities. At the beginning of the 21st century, Howard and Marika Stone (2004), in their book *Too Young to Retire*, argue that 60 or even 65 is too young for retirement. In this book, the entrepreneurial couple provides suggestions for finding new forms of work. Jeri Sedlar and Rick Miners advocate an alternative to retirement in their book, *Don't Retire, REWIRE!* (2003). They suggest that instead of retiring, people should get in touch with their personal key motivators and apply them to new forms of work. All these authors suggest that after leaving a full-time career in an organization, people can tap buried dreams to move out of their organizations and become entrepreneurs.

Renewment

Helen Dennis, a leading researcher into alternative life plans, maintains that retirement, which to her suggests elderly withdrawal, is no longer a viable option for most people. More recently, in *Project Renewment: The First Retirement Model for Career Women*, Dennis and co-author Bernice Bratter (2008), offer a new name for this phase—*renewment*. This term replaces retirement with a word that implies what this phase should be about—life renewal. Dennis argues that whatever name we give this period in our lives, we see it as a time of change—as a journey, not a destination. Her view is particularly appropriate for senior nurses.

At the beginning of the 21st century, we have already moved away from the perception of retirement as a time of not working or as a life of leisure to embrace the paradox of a "working retirement." With all these attempts to change how people view and experience retirement, Americans are clearly in need of clarification, redefinition, experimentation, and invention.

The Future of Retirement in the 21st Century

Several major forces are pushing us toward a new view of retirement.

■ First, people are living so much longer than they did when retirement was institutionalized. Life expectancy now may reach into the 80s and 90s, and even further. Retirement as we've known it just wasn't designed for the longevity revolution that has been changing the life course of millions of people. Instead of lasting just a few years, retirement might stretch for 30 or 40 years; it might last longer than a first career and full-time, gainful employment. On a personal basis, that means you could have more than 20 million minutes on your hands. What are you going to do with all that time? With so much more life to live, people want to create new patterns that are more fulfilling than current views of retirement have envisioned, but social conditions are not favorable. As of yet, we have virtually no institutions or policies that help people plan and prepare for a phase in life as long, and potentially as important and meaningful, as a full-time professional career. Without such needed change, many might experience what Lee Iacocca, the retired automobile executive, did when he confessed, "I flunked retirement."

> "As of yet, we have virtually no institutions or policies that help people plan and prepare for a phase in life as long, and potentially as important and meaningful, as a full-time professional career."

■ Second, when Social Security was inaugurated, the government wanted older workers to give up space in the workforce to younger workers who desperately needed jobs. Today the numbers have been reversed; older people are beginning to outnumber young workers. Some economists and business leaders have already begun to worry about the shortage of replacements for experienced workers in an aging workforce. This fact is particularly troublesome in some industries and professions; health care is clearly at risk. Currently, the health care industry does not have enough physicians, nurses, and technicians to care for a growing population, especially not an aging society. Political and organizational leaders must shift to a different mindset. Organizations need to drastically rethink their employment and leadership strategies to retain the wisdom, experience, skills, and creativity of older workers to meet a critical shortage of employees. This conclusion is particularly relevant to the shortage of nurses. As we shall see in Chapter 6, some nurses are already combining new forms of work with a new approach to retirement management in retirement transition programs.

■ Third, if the large cohort of baby boomers takes retirement at 65 or earlier, the workforce won't contain enough people to contribute to the Social Security bank account, which will be required to pay out a shrinking sum to more retirees. Were this model to prevail, available Social Security funds will diminish by 2040, so retirees at mid-century will not be able to rely on benefits comparable to those available now. However, dire predictions of what will happen to Social Security and a growing cohort of retirees are based on patterns of retirement in the 20th century. If senior workers in their early 60s remain in the workforce longer, thus contributing to Social Security for a longer stretch of time, that bank account could remain solvent and even grow. If more people work past 65 or 70, a different scenario could emerge, and workers in 2040 might wonder what all the worry was about at the turn of the 21st century.

- Fourth, people with longer life expectancy who are still vital, healthy, creative, and productive will want to continue working—though not in the same way they did in their Second Age—because their work provides meaning, rejuvenating challenges, chances to continue learning and build friendships, and income to supplement what they have set aside for complete retirement in their Fourth Age. As noted in the last chapter, some older people have already engaged in new forms of life planning, life management, and work. A growing trend in Third Age Life Planning suggests many more people will follow suit. As part of their new design of life after 50, a growing number of nurses will create Third Age Careers as a significant part of their Third Age Life Portfolios.

All the authors and researchers noted in this book agree: Retirement in the 21st century won't continue to be what it has been in the past. Fifty years ago, retirement was often considered a one-time event, a destination that one should aim for after working. Now, retirement is seen as a process, a journey, a phase in life that is marked by changes. In approaching a retirement that could last for several decades, you should plan to phase into it. More people are delaying retirement, rather than taking early retirement. Most people are taking other forms of work after leaving a full-time career or job. Many people are returning to work after taking retirement. A growing number of people are even resisting the notion of retirement altogether, even if they can afford it. Retirement is an institution that cannot continue in the form it was conceived in the 20th century.

New Forms of Work in a Working Retirement

A trend toward the paradox of "working retirement" has already begun. More older people are working now than just 20 years ago. In 1990 those older than 65 constituted less than 3% of the workforce; that number has increased to 5% and is rising. In 2000, the number of people 65 and older still working was 1 in 5; by 2006 it had already risen to 1 in 4 (Aizeman, 2007). During downturns in the economy, more people postpone retirement to stay in the workforce, because they need income just to keep up. Furthermore, some people who love their careers have continued to work, albeit with greater flexibility and more personal freedom. Today a majority of retirees are seeking employment after leaving a full-time career, either because they need additional income or they need something to fill up empty time.

"Many Americans, perhaps a majority, have not planned ahead carefully enough for full-time retirement that could last for decades."

Rising costs of living are partly responsible for this trend; a decline in savings represents another economic factor. Since the 1960s, average yearly savings for Americans have declined from 10% to 1%. Many Americans, perhaps a majority, have not planned ahead carefully enough for full-time retirement that could last for decades. In interviews, nurses have reported they have not done enough to prepare for a long period of retirement. Increasingly, Americans are postponing retirement after leaving full-time careers by taking jobs that are less challenging and less meaningful than their previous work. These are often seen as temporary or short-term jobs; they are bridges serving an economic and perhaps a social purpose until something better comes along. However, people often hold these positions until they decide to enter retirement on a full-time basis. Professor Joseph Quinn, an economist at Boston College, has been studying this new phenomenon of bridge jobs for more than a decade. According to his book, *Retirement Patterns and Bridge Jobs in the 1990s*, people often remain stuck in bridge jobs because nothing better is available (1999). When baby boomers say they want to work during retirement, a bridge job is not exactly what they have in mind. What surveys have consistently shown is that people thinking about work in their sixth, seventh, or eighth decade are seeking meaning, purpose, social connection, and an opportunity for continued learning, not just a paycheck and a chance to fill an empty slot of time. Senior nurses have expressed the same sentiments. Unfortunately, that kind of opportunity too often is not available, because a cultural lag exists between what older people want and need and possibilities that exist in the workforce.

Encore Careers

Marc Freedman, author and founder of Civic Ventures, not only has provided a withering criticism of conventional retirement, but also more significantly has developed a dramatically different alternative. He has argued that people approaching retirement age need to design a new life that offers greater meaning, challenge, and fulfillment by shifting from chosen careers to a completely different kind of work. His term Encore Career points not to a transitional stage or bridge, but represents "an entire stage of life and work—a destination and a category of work unto itself" (Freedman, 2007, p. 148). Sometimes an Encore Career evolves as a nearly full-time volunteer effort. For example, he cites former executives who leave the corporate world to devote themselves to inner-city schools; a successful car salesman who now helps low income people buy good, inexpensive automobiles; or hospital executives who work with the homeless. Civic Ventures offers annual prizes to outstanding individuals who have made significant social contributions through innovative volunteer commitments. Perhaps of special interest to nurses are volunteer possibilities in health care, such as Samaritan House Clinic in San Mateo, California, or Volunteers in Medicine, a national organization that was started by a retired doctor in Hilton Head, South Carolina, who realized that the low-income workers in his exclusive community did not have health care (Freedman, 1999) .

Freedman has expanded his earlier recommendation of volunteer work so that an Encore Career usually includes a blend of idealism and pragmatism; drawing a salary is important, but so is making a meaningful contribution to society. While contributing to your income, this form of work can include greater flexibility, personal freedom, and a sense of purpose. To some of the people he has studied, it represents the realization of a dream that was suppressed early in life in favor of a conventional career. Freedman recommends that before starting an Encore Career, people should take a sabbatical, where they can rest and become refreshed after decades of hard work. Then with renewed energy and a fresh vision, they can engage in work that really matters. He sees in this proposal a significant social change that transforms retirement, because it encourages people to continue to work in ways that truly use their talents to support the economy as well as themselves. His view represents a drastic departure from Del Webb's vision of a life of leisure in the Golden Years. To Freedman, the possibility that individuals in the second half of life dedicate themselves to service constitutes one of America's great hopes for the future.

This alternative vision addresses the forces that are driving a redefinition of retirement. An Encore Career offers people greater meaning and a sense of purpose lacking in the view of retirement as leisure. It fills out a shrinking workforce and uses talents and wisdom that would otherwise be lost to society. It keeps Social Security solvent, as people continue to contribute to the bank rather than draw on it. An Encore Career also marks a significant advance on the growing popularity of bridge jobs. Unlike the latter, it allows older people to develop a lasting legacy. To realize this possibility requires a great deal of soul searching and ongoing Third Age Life Planning, as described in Chapter 1. Such an alternative might well be a desirable challenge for Third Age nurses to consider, or it could be a choice to enter nursing after 50 when a first career has ended.

Retirement Management

Another alternative has been promoted by William Byham, author, founder, and CEO of Development Dimensions International (DDI), an international company that promotes organizational development, leadership, and human resource management. Byham's vision was presented in his book, *70: The New 50—Retirement Management: Retaining the Energy and Expertise of Experienced Employees* (2007). While not specifically focused on nurses, his model could be applied to hospitals and other health care organizations that need to change if the shortage of nurses is to be solved. In Chapter 6 we shall recommend our own model, **Retirement Transition,** which is similar to his but with a broader scope that includes Third Age Life Planning. Byham approaches the idea of retirement from the vantage point of demographics—companies cannot afford to lose the wisdom and expertise of talented, experienced, knowledgeable leaders and employees, because the 78 million baby boomers cannot be adequately replaced by the 40 million people of Generation X. In the 21st century, companies need baby boomers to keep working, and baby boomers have indicated they want to continue working, though not necessarily to the same extent or in the same way. Byham lists a variety of reasons why organizations should reconsider their human resources policies to enable them to retain older workers rather than lose them to retirement:

"Retirement management means a long, carefully planned transition into retirement, one that is fully supported by a company."

- Older workers have knowledge and experience valuable to the company.

- They can fill hard to replace positions.

- They can keep positions filled until backup can be found and trained.

- Retaining them reduces costs of recruitment.

- Retention meets older workers' financial needs.

- Keeping people in the workforce preserves the viability of Social Security (Byham, 2007, pp. 31–32).

All of his reasons apply to the situation of health care and the need to retain senior nurses to address critical shortages. So does his list of advantages for keeping older workers, which includes:

- Good work habits.

- Loyalty to the organization with few absences.

- Fully engaged in their work.

- Perform as well as or better than younger workers.

- Better at communication, taking initiative, assuming responsibility.

- More engaged in planning, organizational leadership, and sustaining organizational culture (Byham, 2007, pp. 80–82).

Byham's argument is more suitable to hospitals than the two previous models of bridge jobs and Encore Careers. To address the needs of organizations as well as older workers, Byham has developed a distinctive view of *retirement management*. By this term he means a long, carefully planned transition into retirement, one that is fully supported by a company. Such a transition could last a few years, or it could last more than a decade. He recommends that administrators be flexible in their approaches to retirement; recognize the value older workers can add to strategy, operations, and company culture; and offer financial planning and coaching to assist workers as they transition toward retirement at a later date. For example, organization administrators can provide leaders and employees with workshops and coaches to help them with life and financial planning. They might also change their pay schedules by compensating transitioning employees according to their contributions, instead of buying them out with retirement plans. If people are paid relative to their contributions and given the choice between working and not working, many older workers might accept less money for doing less work or less demanding work. Byham (2007) points out that new laws under the Employee Retirement Income Security Act (ERISA) make customizing transition-to-retirement pay legal. Furthermore, as people switch from defined benefits pensions to defined contribution pensions, they can begin to draw from the latter to supplement their income.

In addition to helping leaders and employees design employment plans to retain their valued contributions, administrators should support new ventures for older workers. For example, they should consider putting them in new positions on a full- or part-time basis, allowing them to pursue new forms of work that are compatible with their values and emerging interests. Seasoned workers can become mentors to new hires, take on a special assignment requiring valuable knowledge, fill in for people on leave or special assignments, or teach new hires how to contribute to planning or develop their leadership. Chapter 6 reports on a few innovative hospitals where this kind of approach has already occurred.

These strategies add significant value to both organizations and individuals, and at the same time reduce costs. It is much less costly to retain a valued employee than it is to search for and train a replacement. Besides reducing costs, this kind of organizational flexibility also yields increased productivity and retention of valued leaders and employees.

> "It is much less costly to retain a valued employee than it is to search for and train a replacement."

In spite of the social, economic, and organizational benefits that retirement management offers, it has not yet become a recognized change movement. Still, some leading business organizations have been moving in this direction. Deloitte Consulting has established flexible career planning within its organization; it now allows its leaders to customize their jobs, choosing how many hours to put in, where, and on which projects. Aerospace Corporation has allowed older workers to downscale to part-time work or to self-employed consulting status; the company even allows full-time employees to take a leave up to 3 months each year. John Deere has retained a small cadre of workers in their 70s who work with flexible schedules that better fit their life plans. Other organizations such as Home Depot give older workers the option to change location during the year—summers in New England, winters in Florida. CVS/pharmacy and Borders bookstore have policies that call for a workforce consisting of 20-30% older workers, who have more flexibility in their schedules. We can expect to see this trend expand to become a norm, rather than an exception, in the 21st century. Chapter 6 shows how some nurses and hospitals are already developing retirement transitions that allow senior nurses—in their 60s and 70s—to keep working past retirement age in new ways.

Byham provides a survey of what older workers are looking for in their retirement management programs. Although nurses apparently were not included in this survey, his findings are very similar to views expressed by nurses. Older workers in general who consider continuing to work in their organizations want to:

- Ease into retirement, not enter it abruptly as a singular event

- Have more personal time

- Have the opportunity to help others in their work

- Work not so hard nor so much, with flexible workloads

- Have more vacation time

- Have the option of cycling in and out of work

What might these new work schedules look like? A rich variety of possibilities exists. Some older workers have requested working 3 days, with 7 days off, or working 3, 10-hour days each week. Others have requested working a full schedule for 3 to 12 months and then having 6 months off. After the rigid expectation of a 40-hour work week for an entire year is lifted, you have nearly as many possibilities as individuals to take advantage of these changes.

How can older workers pay for such reduced workloads? They have to start planning for a long transition into retirement years earlier. However, assuming they have been contributing to defined contribution pension funds and 401(k)s, older workers can begin to take systematic withdrawals from these funds while still contributing to them. That way, pension funds remain in effect for them to draw upon when they eventually enter retirement full-time. Also, after older workers reach full retirement age (this ranges from 66, for workers born in 1943 to 1954, to 67, for those born in 1960 and later; see www.ssa.gov/pubs/retirechart.htm for specifics), they can draw the full amount of their Social Security. Byham shows that his alternative transition strategy is affordable, making full retirement a realistic financial possibility later in life. It is a win/win proposition, providing desired forms of work for older workers who have been identified by management as necessary for organizational success. This kind of transformation of retirement also offers great hope for America's future—and especially for nurses.

Third Age Careers for Nurses

So far, three alternatives to the American norm of retirement have been presented:

1. Leaving jobs to start a new, income-producing career as an entrepreneur or taking a bridge job

2. Leaving jobs to design totally new Encore Careers, which serve the public good and can be accomplished either as a volunteer or with some income

3. Continuing in one's company, but in a different mode, by designing a retirement management transition within the organization

For an optimum outcome, all of these require that nurses engage in sustained Third Age Life Planning. With the first two options, individuals launch out on their own; the third option calls for collaborative organizational planning and support. This latter option might be most appropriate for nurses who want to remain in health care, particularly in hospitals, but who want to continue nursing in ways more compatible with their experience, changing interests, and needs. Focus-group interviews conducted by a Holy Names University School of Nursing team reported in the next chapter clearly demonstrate senior nurses' desire to reduce physical work, back-to-back shifts, excessive paperwork, and so on. Instead, senior nurses said they wanted to contribute their knowledge and wisdom in health care as mentors, teachers, public relations officers, and leaders. For all alternatives to conventional retirement, the initiative must start with the individual, who begins by asking basic Third Age questions, such as:

- Where do I want to go next?

- Who do I want to become?

- What is most important?

- What do I value?

- What new elements do I want to add or recover?

It's time for a course change. As Schofield has put it, after 50, it's up to us to discover and decide what direction we want to take (Schofield, 2007).

Redefining Work

In Chapter 1, we discussed how to redesign life after 50 for an emerging personal identity by building a Third Age Life Portfolio. A life portfolio organizes a variety of chosen interests and activities, providing people with a sense of freedom, purpose, and balance that is increasingly important as they grow older. In designing a life portfolio, we need to include some form of work that expresses who we are becoming and gives us meaning. In the Holy Names University interviews, the vast majority of nurses expressed a love of their work and ambivalence about leaving it in retirement. Even if they could afford retirement, they would consider remaining an active nurse, but they don't want to continue working in the same way. A major objective of this book is to encourage nurses to rethink retirement and consider redesigning their work and their lives.

"A major objective is to encourage nurses to rethink retirement and consider redesigning their work and their lives."

English business writer Charles Handy has a vision of work in the 21st century that supports what nurses have asked for. He maintains that as the nature of work changes, especially in the Third Age, we have *"the chance to shape our work to suit the way we want to live instead of always living to fit in with our work"* (1990, p. 179). His view is especially appropriate to nurses as they consider retirement and possible approaches or alternatives:

> Leisure only makes sense when it is the other side of work, when it is re-creation for more work. Work, I am sure, is what we will want to do, work rediscovered, work redefined to mean more than selling your time to someone else, work that is more in tune with the rest of life, work that is more personal, more creative, more fun. … First of all, we (should) start redefining "work" so that it no longer means only a job. … Our human instincts make us want to contribute to our world, to be useful, and to matter in some way to

other people, to have a reason to get up in the morning. Put that way, work is the purpose of life; it also gives us a pattern or structure for our days, and a chance to meet new people. Purpose, pattern, and people—the three P's at the heart of life (Handy, pp. 180-181).

The task of redefining work within a life portfolio often calls for designing a *Third Age Career*. Just what does that mean and what does it entail? The term *career* originally meant a racecourse. As it applies to our work, it often still implies racing ahead toward some goal: income, promotion, position, recognition, influence, or status. A person's Second Age career usually has a linear direction. We speak of career ladders—one starts at the bottom and moves up, one step at a time. To transition to a Third Age Career, we take a direction that opens like a starburst—an unfolding of creativity that expresses our passion, purpose, talents, knowledge and wisdom; a set of core values; and a sense of fun. This new pattern of work begins by redefining work not as a job but as an expression of who we are, what we want to contribute, how we want to find meaning, and what legacy we want to leave to our world. This new pattern of work should fit with and support the design we bring to our unfolding lives.

As they tracked dozens of people who have creatively designed their Third Age lives, Sadler and Krefft discovered a rich variety of ways people are shaping Third Age Careers (2008). The previous chapter introduced several of them. Susan left a career with a bank to start her own consulting company, where she was free to center on the feminine values that became the core of her life. Her Third Age Careers included working for pay and volunteering, helping women clarify their visions and start new enterprises. Rebecca left her career as a merchandising manager in her husband's company to launch a new career as a fine artist. That work became her passion and also allowed her to express who she was becoming. Ted designed his Third Age Career while continuing to work for the same architectural firm he had been with for more than 40 years. He negotiated terms for a new form of work that allowed him to put in only 20 to 30 hours a week, with great flexibility to allow for traveling to sites and to focus on his personal interests. In addition, he could branch out to develop new careers, such as teaching architecture and working with local governments to redesign urban landscapes. He also became more involved in volunteer work, focusing on environmental design and conservation.

These people experienced greater satisfaction and fulfillment as they shifted into new life/work patterns. Personal fulfillment is a major reason why nurses should consider changing course into Third Age Career planning.

"Personal fulfillment is a major reason why nurses should consider changing course into Third Age Career planning."

Another man's story from the research of Sadler and Krefft illustrates a pattern that could easily be relevant to many nurses who are interested in changing the course of their careers in hospitals. Dan worked in life insurance his entire career, moving up from salesman to district manager. He was successful in his work, enjoyed his job, and liked his clients and colleagues. He had experienced a strong sense of purpose in his work, but as he reached 60, he felt confused. He wasn't sure where he wanted to go next. After some counseling, reading, and considerable reflection, he concluded he just had to "pull the plug" on his career. Within a few months, he retired from the company and went off with several buddies for a long bike trip in Europe. He had no plans and no clear ideas of what to do next. He returned home after 3 months, and the company came calling. His boss told him they needed to fill a yet-to-be-designed position to help the company address radical changes in the market. He had experience, a sense of the company's strengths and distinctive qualities, and the connections they needed to expand into different markets. In essence, they offered Dan the chance to shape his work the way he wanted to live and to serve the company in ways that nobody else could. After a year, at the age of 62, Dan reported he was thrilled with his new life, the challenge and satisfaction of his work, and the future direction he was carving out as an alternative to retirement. His Third Age Career was every bit as rewarding and challenging as his Second Age Career; in addition, he had more free time to spend with his wife, family, friends, and in volunteer activities. This alternative to retirement was an opportunity for personal growth, for learning, for leadership development, for increasing his sense of meaning and purpose, and for having more fun. He did not give up on the idea of retirement; he just saw the long transition as a fulfilling journey until he was ready for retirement, whatever that might mean when he gets there (Sadler & Krefft, 2008). Many nurses can also redesign their careers within a hospital setting or another health care organization, if their company provides the kind of assistance, creative planning, and support that leaders in the life insurance company invented for Dan.

Taking Steps Toward a Third Age Career

As nurses begin designing a portfolio life, here are some steps they can take to give shape to a Third Age Career:

"Nurses need to recover a sense of dignity and purpose that is inherent in professional work."

- **Realize that work is more than a job.** The term *job* comes from a different era, the Industrial Revolution, where work was designed around machines, and where people were given narrowly defined, measurable tasks to perform in conformance to the requirements of machines and mechanistic bureaucracies. Especially with the development of professions and an Information Age, human endeavors are more greatly appreciated and needed. Nurses need to recover a sense of dignity and purpose that is inherent in professional work.

- **Free yourself for what is important.** In the Third Age, nurses need to rediscover the ideals that brought them into nursing in the first place. Now is the time to clarify and reaffirm core values and to affirm what matters most in your life—and in your work.

- **Dig deep, let go, and experiment.** Third Age Life Planning calls for an inward journey, to get in touch with yourself and the person you want to become as you grow older. In affirming this new self, you need to let go of activities and habits that don't fit and can hinder progress with that emerging model. To chart a new course, you need to experiment with new behaviors, new interests, and new ways of doing what you have done for so many years.

- **In this experimentation, do work that matters.** Doing work that matters requires not only clarifying what matters to you, but negotiating with your organization so that you and other Third Age nurses can focus on mutually agreed upon activities, commitments, and requirements.

- **Redefine success.** The model of success in the Second Age was largely composed of extrinsic measures: income, promotion, recognition, and influence. In the Third Age, you need to define success more in terms that are inherently meaningful. Make a contribution. Leave a legacy. Do the work you love, and love what you do. Success might mean engaging in the process in which you increasingly realize unique potential, make a contribution to people you care about, and experience more *flow* in your evolving life.

- **Balance work and play; balance work and love; balance work that needs to be done with what you want to do.** Find more moments in which your soul sings.

Planning Your Retirement Transition

This chapter has emphasized how retirement for people older than 50 has been changing in the last decade. It no longer represents a one-time event in the life course. Rather, for most people it has become a process of change, with many different shapes, phases, and meanings. Furthermore, full retirement is no longer an aspired destination for healthy, youthful people in their 6th, 7th, or even 8th decade. More and more people are postponing full retirement; the authors of this book are among them. Increasingly, people are phasing into a personally designed lifestyle in a retirement transition. For most nurses and health care institutions, this movement toward retirement transition is good news. Chapter 6 reports on how a few hospitals have already started a formal phased retirement program, one that supports the growth and development of senior nurses, keeps them in the system, and contributes to the improvement of patient care.

With the expansion of the life course and a vital Third Age, we have more time to prepare for an eventual retirement, perhaps later in our Fourth Age (roughly after 75). We have argued that this preparation calls for both Third Age Life Planning and financial planning. Until now many, if not most, people have entered retirement without adequate preparation. They have not thought enough about a dramatic change in their lives; they have not planned how they could live to experience fulfillment and realize their potential, which is really what "the pursuit of happiness" means. Furthermore, they have not anticipated how much income they will need to sustain a desired lifestyle, nor how to draw upon savings and retirement plans to pay their bills. So nurses, along with millions of others, need to mindfully engage in a long-term personal strategy, a longevity strategy, using both Third Age Life Planning and long-term financial planning to guide them through a long transition into retirement.

How can nurses get started? A major objective of this book is to help nurses do the initial work in their personal life planning, but it is only a start. Sadler and Krefft (2008) found that all the people who were successfully redesigning their Third Age lives had assistance from mentors, personal coaches, counselors or therapists, friends, spouses, and organizational leaders. So in addition to what we read and think, most of us need a guide. If an organization is not supporting personal development for Third Age nurses to move into retirement transition, nurses should team up and ask it to begin doing so. If you belong to a union, and its policies are not supportive of this long-term planning for retirement transition, ask it to change policies. However, more immediately, nurses can access a growing network of personal life coaches who specialize in Third Age Life Planning. We have included some resources in the appendix at the end of this book to help you get started. You can also consult with The Center for Third Age Nurses at Holy Names University in Oakland, California. The center is developing an information base and services (learn more at http://www.hnu.edu/hnuNews/centerThirdAge.html).

Second, most nurses need financial help in planning their retirement transition. If the hospital administration does not yet offer such assistance, external financial planners are readily available. Nurses need to describe the changes in their imagined lifestyles and indicate the amount of money needed to support them. If they haven't already done so, they should begin a systematic routine of saving for retirement, contributing as much as is realistically affordable to a pension plan, 401(k), or other retirement account. Ten percent of one's income might be a good place to start. Because financial and investment planning is a foreign field to most professionals, nurses need professional assistance that is trustworthy and reliable for the long term. Help is available. The Center for Third Age Nurses has found the SecurePath program offered by insurance company Transamerica (www.securepathbytransamerica.com), to be dependable. It offers holistic retirement planning that complements the Third Age Life Planning described in this book. If people have not been investing in their future adequately, it is not too late to begin. The change of course in a new direction is already underway. Talk with family, friends, colleagues, and officers in your organization to link up with the people who can help you move in a desired direction right now.

References

Aizeman, N. C. (2007, September 12). Editorial. *The Washington Post,* p. A10.

Bratter, B., & Dennis, H. (2008). *Project renewment: The first retirement model for career women.* New York: Scribner.

Byham, W. C. (2007). *70: The new 50: Retirement management.* Pittsburgh, PA: DDI Press.

Dennis, H. (2001). The new retirement. In W. Zinke & S. Totttershall (Eds.), *Working through demographic change* (pp. 73-80). Boulder, CO: Human Resources Services.

Erikson, E., & Erikson, J. (1986). *Vital involvement in old age.* New York: Norton.

Freedman, M. (1999). *Prime time: How baby boomers will revolutionize retirement and transform America.* New York: Public Affairs.

Freedman, M. (2007). *Encore: Finding work that matters in the second half of life.* New York: Public Affairs.

Giandrea, M., Cahill, K., & Quinn, J. (2007, May 30). *An update on bridge jobs: The HRS war babies.* Retrieved December 11, 2008, from http://fmwww.bc.edu/EC-P/WP670.pdf

Handy, C. (1990). *The age of unreason.* Cambridge, MA: Harvard Business School Press.

Quinn, J. (1999). *Retirement patterns and bridge jobs in the 1990s.* Washington, D.C.: Employee Benefit Research Institute.

Sadler, W.A , & Krefft, J. H. (2008). *Changing course: Navigating life after 50.* Centennial, CO: The Center for Third Age Leadership Press.

Schofield, G. H. (2007). *After 50 it's up to us.* Fort Bragg, CA: Clarity Group.

Sedlar, J., & Miners, R. (2003) *Don't retire, REWIRE! 5 steps to fulfilling work that fuels your passion, suits your personality, or fills your pockets.* Indianapolis, IN: Alpha Books.

Stone, M., & Stone, H. (2004). *Too young to retire.* New York: Penguin Group.

Third Age Nurses | II

Nurses in the Third Age | **3**

Like many things associated with the baby boomer generation, the retirement of nurses could have a lasting and devastating effect. In 2007, the American Hospital Association predicted that unfilled nursing vacancies could reach 1 million by 2010 as nurses in the baby boomer generation retire (Freedman, 2007).

One response to this potential looming crisis is to retain retirement-age nurses in the workforce. But what do nurses want or need for themselves? It turns out that many retirement-age nurses want and need to stay in nursing, but they want their work to be in a form that's physically sustainable and emotionally rewarding and that can support them and their family.

The Facts

According to a report commissioned by the Robert Wood Johnson Foundation (Hatcher, Bleich, Connolly, Davis, Hewlett, & Hill, 2006), of the nurses expressing an interest in working more years, economic factors were the most important affecting retention, but non-economic factors were nearly as important. Work schedules need to be more flexible and balanced. For example, shift work makes work/life balance difficult, and long hours of demanding work contribute to burnout. Scheduling, it seems, needs to be creatively designed, allowing nurses more personal time and more opportunity for control over how they work. New positions and opportunities need to be created that allow nurses to educate and mentor others so they can share what they have spent a lifetime learning.

The report suggested a need for new career paths that can lead to transitioning into retirement. They also stated a need for the development of organizational cultures that are more supportive of nurses and transitions into different forms of work. They noted nurses frequently report feeling undervalued, overworked, and overly controlled. Nurses want more control over their work, opportunities to make and share in important decision-making, greater recognition, more opportunities to make a significant difference in health care, and a clearer focus on doing the work they love and/or on learning new modes of caring (Hatcher et al., 2006).

In addition, the report recommended the following considerations:

- The creation of new positions of responsibility, allowing nurses to expand into preceptor, mentor, best-practice coach, and other role-model positions to educate and support new staff nurses.

- The addition of facilitators for the education of new methods and the learning of new technologies to help older nurses learn and develop new skills.

- The development of seasoned nurses who can make ideal health care system consultants, community liaisons, public relations officers, relief nurses, safety officers, patient educators, and nursing faculty.

The Center for Third Age Nurses

In light of this and similar evidence pointing to the need to retain this population of highly trained and valuable nurses in the profession, the Center for Third Age Nurses was launched at Holy Names University in Oakland, California, in order to study the issues and create programs and processes that could support nurses in the Third Age. Through this endeavor, the authors of this book became involved in providing information, education, and other help for nurses interested in staying in the workforce.

Early discussions during the development of the Center focused on the need to learn about the problems and/or expectations of Third Age nurses. Those discussions led to the development of three strategies:

1. Conduct focus groups of Third Age nurses so they could learn about their interests, concerns, and career goals.

2. Create workshops based on what was learned from focus group feedback.

3. Develop educational programs to help Third Age nurses make careful and useful decisions about their future careers.

Third Age Focus Groups

Early in the fall of 2007, the first focus group of nurses from various hospitals and public health agencies was convened at the Center. Six other groups of nurses were assembled over the next 6 months until more than 250 nurses had participated in these focus groups.

The Questions

The same list of questions was offered to each group, and each group was assured of confidentiality. That is, the participants were told the results of their discussion would be shared only as a group response. They were also told the purpose of the discussions was not to reach consensus, that different opinions were encouraged, and that the importance of those different opinions would be acknowledged. Each session lasted about 1 1/2 hours. The list of questions included the following:

- In one sentence, describe what you like about nursing.

- If you could change one thing in nursing today, what would it be?

- The Third Age Task Force is exploring the possibility of using retired nurses in some capacity, given the extent of the nursing shortage. What are your thoughts about such an idea?

- If such an idea were to materialize, what would be an essential element for you to consider participation?

- What problems, if any, do you see with the idea?

- What do you see as the best way to find retired nurses? And what criteria, if any, should be applied to their selection?

- How do you think we could best utilize the talents and experiences of retired nurses?

- One area of need in nursing today is for clinical faculty. Would you be interested in pursuing this avenue? What resources would you need to help you pursue this option?

- What haven't we asked that you would like to share or would like the Center to know about?

The Answers

Three strong themes became evident from the responses. These themes were:

1. **Nurses love their work.** Even at the end of a career, nurses still loved nursing, but most were weary of what they were doing. They wanted to end that aspect of their career, but they did not know how to begin making changes. They offered comments such as "I love serving people," "I like helping people feel responsible for their own health," "I like seeing people get better," "I love empowering people to seize control of their lives," "I like teaching people about how to stay well," "I like working with students."

2. **Most nurses need to keep working after 50 for financial reasons.** While they knew they needed to "make a living," they were unsure about how that would look or where it could be accomplished if they left the position they currently occupied.

3. **Nurses seek collaborative environments.** Over and over again the nurses talked about the wisdom and skill they had acquired over time, yet they did not know what to do with it given the present-day delivery care models and the lack of collaboration and acknowledgement of their talents. They suggested being a mentor; working in the community with children/teenagers; being an advocate; counseling high school students about the best way to seek and accomplish a career in nursing; teaching students in colleges/universities about the aspects of the discipline that are missing, such as respect for cultural differences; helping to make the workforce of nurses more diverse through culture, ethnicity, and religion to better match the demographics of the patient population; and many other needed and valuable strategies.

> "Even at the end of a career, nurses still loved nursing, but most were weary of what they were doing."

The concepts of commitment and engagement were recurring themes during the focus-group sessions. The nurses were committed to helping others and they wanted to stay engaged in some fashion, even though they were unclear about what that meant.

A qualitative researcher analyzed the data and concluded that RNs in the study:

- Think about ways to stay role-engaged that are consistent with personal interest—meaning, they were not clouded by sentiment but instead put themselves first in order of priority.

- Envision ways to use their wisdom and experience in a meaningful way.

- Recognize barriers exist to achieving the right fit for staying engaged.

- Actively participate in thinking about how to stay engaged, but do not know what to do about it.

- See a focus on Third Age as a valuable way to increase awareness of opportunities and facilitation transition.

- Believe others could benefit from Third Age information.

- Think pursuing Third Age Career planning is a viable way to help facilitate and support commitment/engagement.

The Recommendations

These nurses realized there are few paying jobs that exist for the pursuit of these avenues of engagement. They also realized most of them were not politically astute about the ways to implement their ideas. Few belonged to any professional organization or even knew the name of their senators or congressman. They devised this list of recommendations:

1. In order to stay committed and engaged, attention must be given to three activities:

   ▪ Link personal goals with employment options.

   ▪ Promote work as an opportunity to express passion for nursing.

   ▪ Align and create a position and place to match personal goals and passion for nursing.

2. Explore new options and disseminate the information to others.

3. Continue opportunities to dialogue on the issue.

4. Increase awareness of the issues and needs.

5. Pursue Center ideas to facilitate and support Third Age nurses' desires or continued role-engagement commitment.

When it came to the identification of barriers that might dissuade them from becoming further involved in nursing, nurses quickly identified two:

1. Time

2. Ignorance

Even though the nurses felt "burned out" in their present job, they were so busy trying to keep up with the demands of the position with the current shortage of nurses, that they had no time to consider something else. In fact, they thoroughly enjoyed the opportunity to discuss the questions set forth by the facilitators, because it gave them time to think about their work lives and even to consider something else. However, they also felt ignorant about what else they could do and

"The nurses were overjoyed when they learned *retirement* was a dead word, that they could find life after their current job, and that they need not be burdened by the concept of *work*."

even what else was available to them as a nurse. Many also felt out of touch with current technology—computers, personal digital assistants (PDAs), robotic surgery, etc. In fact, many were insecure about being seen as "incompetent" or "stupid." They urged the staff of the Center to keep them informed and to continue with the development of services for Third Age nurses. They made it clear they needed help with planning for the next step in their professional lives.

Workshops for Third Age Nurses

The second strategy was to use what was learned from the focus groups to offer help to Third Age nurses interested in their future career. Workshops were designed and are being offered to accomplish this task. Workshops are valuable because they provide a way to determine the validity of the questions and needs of nurses. They also provide a venue for helping nurses make vital decisions about their future career.

Two skills are presented at these workshops: the Six Principles of Growth and Renewal, and Designing a Third Age Life Portfolio. The Six Principles of Growth and Renewal were explored in Chapter 1 and include:

- Practicing mindful reflection and risk-taking

- Developing realistic optimism

- Building a positive Third Age identity

- Redefining and balancing work and play

- Balancing greater freedom and deeper, more intimate relationships

- Caring for others, earth, and self

Each principle is explained, and then the nurses are asked to pursue a set of questions to accomplish each principle. For example, with principle one, group members are asked to consider who they really are and to determine the ways they can be that person. After a time to complete this reflection, the group members share their discoveries.

Similar strategies are used as each nurse learns how to build a life portfolio based on the data generated from the six principles. (Note, an in-depth discussion of the six principles of renewal and the strategies for building a life portfolio can be found in Chapter 1 of this text.)

Workshop Outcomes

The outcomes of the workshops are many. In most instances, nurses are astounded when they learn what they can do and that others have the same concerns. In fact, one of most valuable outcomes from the workshops is the chance nurses of the Third Age have to meet others of the Third Age who have similar needs and concerns about their future work life. In fact, they were overjoyed when they learned "retirement" is a dead word, that there is a life after their current job, and that they need not be burdened by the concept of "work." All of these issues are discussed in the workshops as they have been presented in this book. This discussion has given many a new and exciting vision of the future.

Another valuable outcome of the workshops is the nurses' interest in having a place where they can get help, support, and direction. Until very recently, there has been no place for people reaching retirement age to get information, resources, or referrals for the next period of their lives. The Center for Third Age Nurses is exactly what they need and want. The Center continues to plan for more services to support nurses in this age group. Further, involvement in these workshops elevates the participants' view of themselves as, until recently, growing older has not been valued. In fact, many nurses do not tell their age for fear of being isolated, put down, or kept from advancing. Just having the opportunity to learn about the changes across the country and around the world about the newest conceptualization of growing older gives them a lift and improves their self-image.

Another distinguishing aspect of the workshops is the way the content and activities are organized. For example, participants are organized into mixed groups by age, nursing specialty, geographic area, and workplace. When they are allowed to select a group, they tend to sit with friends and do not get as involved or learn as much about other perspectives. Another aspect of importance when conducting a workshop is the ratio of facilitator to group members. Generally small groups—at most six nurses—work best, for the nurses are more likely to participate when the group is small. The content is organized such that information is presented with follow-up activities, so the participants will not "tune out." Sometimes the small group work is shared, and sometimes it is kept confidential. This all depends on the nature of the subject. For example, the nurses usually have no difficulty sharing ideas about what they want; on the other hand, information generated about their identity is usually kept private, unless the nurse wants to share. Generally, as the day progresses and the nurses get to know each other, they become more interested in sharing everything.

Other Sources of Information

"Facing retirement is no longer the only option for nurses reaching 50 and beyond."

Facing retirement is no longer the only option for nurses reaching 50 and beyond. The options for continued involvement in the workforce are many, and the desire to continue to be involved is incredible, both because of need and because of desire.

A close examination of the current health care system and how it has changed over the last 50 years, with the introduction of technology and increased patient awareness of their health problems, suggests nurses, particularly older nurses, must be ready, prepared, and motivated for change.

References

Byham, W. C. (2007). *70: The new 50: Retirement management*. Pittsburgh, PA: DDI Press.

Freedman, M. (2007). *Encore: Finding work that matters in the second half of life*. New York: Public Affairs.

Hatcher, B., Bleich, M. R., Connolly, C., Davis, K., Hewlett, P. O., & Hill, K. S. (2006). *Wisdom at work: The importance of the older and experienced nurse in the workplace*. Princeton, NJ: Robert Woods Johnson Foundation.

Planning for Nursing Fulfillment in the Third Age Years | 4

It's never too early to begin planning your Third Age transition. Toward that goal, the Center for Third Age Nurses has created activities to help nurses transition into their Third Age. The following activities are the result of the work of the Center and its members.

7 Activities for Getting Ready to Make a Career Change

Activity 1: Prepare a Plan—A Life Portfolio—for the Future

Don't wait to ask the question "What can I do now?" after reaching retirement age or when your body has made bedside work impossible. According to Michelle Paolucci Peebles, RN, MSN, in her 2008 *Nursing Spectrum* article, "Journey to Jobs: Promising Paths for Nurses," nurses at the beginning of their career need to look forward and plan the pathway they want to pursue as a professional. The day nurses become licensed is the perfect time to start thinking about where that license can and will take them and what additional training and education they will need to achieve their eventual goals. Planning for advanced nursing education early can open up many mid- and late-life options, including:

- Teaching

- Nurse practitioner work

- Public and/or community health nursing

- Opportunities in acute care settings, particularly with technology and hospital Magnet™ initiatives

- Business-based roles outside of traditional health care operations

"Seeing age as a positive and not a negative can help you catch up in the planning process."

Preparing a life portfolio is a good way to plan the future. While it may sound counter-intuitive, early career and "retirement" planning actually increases flexibility, allowing quick and easy career redirection, a variety of career experiences, or time off in mid-career for family care or volunteer, missionary, or other work. Also, it allows you to be the one making decisions in the Third Age and beyond. For example, many nurses begin their career on a medical-surgical unit, progress to a specialty unit, and then go into the community, whether as a visiting nurse, palliative care nurse, nurse practitioner, or community/public health nurse. Some move into faculty positions and non-clinical health care work, such as with design/architectural firms and drug and insurance companies, just to name a few. Nurses are often sought by businesses that serve the health care industry because the largest customers of these industries frequently are hospitals. Few professionals know hospitals better than nurses.

Being educationally prepared early for any of these positions fosters credibility and allows for choice when a nurse's physical or other circumstances demand a change. Many nurses love bedside care, but time and age can change that perspective. Frequently, for nurses past age 40, the back and legs cannot provide the support needed to care for bedridden patients.

Seeing age as a positive and not a negative can help you catch up in the planning process. Whereas it is better to plan early, it is never too late to start. The first activity is to prepare a life portfolio. According to Sadler and Krefft (2008), four principles must be followed as the portfolio is designed:

- Diversify the flow of your life

- Free yourself for what's important

- Create the right space

- Live vitally

(See Chapter 1 for an in-depth discussion of the way to develop a life portfolio).

Activity 2: Know Your Strengths

Many people do not know their strengths. Nurses are certainly not the only group that does not take the time to inventory the characteristics that propel their successes and their failures. Taking the time to identify your strengths is critical to understanding your options. See Table 1 for a way to identify your strengths.

Strengths	Weaknesses
Patient	Impatient
Perseverant	Lack fortitude
Flexible	Inflexible
Approachable	Unapproachable
Friendly	Ascerbic/unkind
Organized	Disorganized

Strengths	Weaknesses
Punctual	Perpetually late
Responsible	Irresponsible
Accountable	Blames others
Respectful	Disrespectful
Timely	Time waster
Risk Taker	Hesitant or fearful of risk

"If you know your strengths, that awareness creates a cadre of tools you can use to help define and build your career pathway."

It really doesn't matter what the strengths are; what counts is that you are aware of your strengths so you can use the strengths when needed and ensure the weaknesses are under control or do not lead you into trouble.

An important aspect of knowing your strengths is having an awareness that they can change given your situation, your needs, and your age. One nurse told a story about how her strengths as a young nurse were being flexible and open to others' ideas. As she grew older and gained a variety of experiences, she added strengths that eventually included being a risk taker, being a team player, being well-prepared for new experiences, and being a leader. Time and experience helped her build a greater array of strengths.

Significantly, if you know your strengths, that awareness creates a cadre of tools you can use to help define and build your career pathway. This helps you when an opportunity arises in which you need to make a decision. If the opportunity fits your defined strengths, then your decision is easier.

Activity 3: Evaluate Your Needs

Just as it's important to know your strengths, it is important to know your needs. Unlike strengths, *needs* are often dependent on the circumstances at the time or are affected by the situation. For example, if your situation requires you to be available at different times and in different ways, then flexibility in a position is needed. This could mean finding a position, like a job in the community, where the hours are flexible because they are defined by the nurse rather then by the institution. On the other hand, if being organized is a requisite for a specific job or event, then being able to pull things together in an organized fashion is needed. For instance, being a nurse manager, where there are many variables to manage and many people to supervise, would mean the nurse would need substantial organizational skills.

One of the most obvious needs for being able to function in the Third Age is to know what jobs/positions are available and what you need to qualify for what is available. It is a two-fold need; it is a combination of knowing what is out there, that is, what the workforce needs are, and whether you have the education, experience, or qualifications for the position.

Many nurses do not take advantage of educational opportunities until late in their careers, and then they are unsure what to pursue and where to pursue it. Often the biggest need for Third Age nurses is advanced educational preparation, but nurses frequently claim to be too old to return to school. But this isn't true. Getting over this idea might be one of the biggest hurdles nurses face. For example, a 55-year-old nurse recently completed a BSN degree and was able to receive funding for a MSN degree. She hesitated going on for the MSN because of her age, until she learned from a 60-year-old colleague that she had done so and had acquired a high-paying position because of the advanced degree. The 55-year-old went on to acquire the advanced degree.

An equally important need is to know trends in the health care industry and what future opportunities may be presented as systems change. One of the most common complaints Third Age nurses express is being unaware of what is happening within health care outside their specific job and what changes are coming up. Thus, the need for future thinking and staying informed is an important one. Third Age nurses need to know about:

- Technology changes, such as the electronic medical record.

- Situation-Background-Assessment-Recommendation (SBAR), a method for communication.

- Robotic surgery, that is, surgery performed by small robotic instruments at the direction of the surgeon.

- Telemedicine, which is health care provided by a professional at one location to a patient at a different location via interactive television.

- Healing environments.

- Family Focused Care.

Clearly knowing your needs is as important as knowing your strengths, as one tends to affect the other. If you know your needs, then you can assess your strengths to see if they can help you meet your needs. And, vice versa, if you know your strengths, then you can work on using them to determine your needs. Once you have determined what you can offer, a look at the health care system and what is needed is appropriate. The goal is to match your needs with the needs of the workplace.

Activity 4: Prepare Yourself for the Future

Just as it is important to identify strengths and needs, it is also important to think ahead, particularly if you want to change your career path.

Thinking ahead also demands keeping in touch with change in your profession and your particular specialty area within the industry. To do so means being a member of a professional organization, reading the current nursing literature, keeping abreast of daily news, and keeping current with the local health care issues. While Web technology such as blogs, Really Simple Syndication (RSS) feeds, and e-newsletter subscriptions can seem daunting, learning to be a savvy consumer of technology can help you more easily keep up. Most organizations offer free RSS feeds from their Web pages, and many other organizations offer e-newsletters. Plan some time in your day to look over these feeds or newsletters, and it won't seem as overwhelming. Resources such as iGoogle (www.igoogle.com) offer free Web-feed aggregators, basically making a one-stop shop to manage and organize all the data you need. If you're uncomfortable with the technology, ask for help. Young people make some of the best teachers for using the technology to the best of its abilities.

> Janet, a nurse, wanted to leave the acute care setting because she was finding it difficult to keep pace with the demands of the job. She thought about doing community health nursing. Unfortunately, when she inquired about the position, she discovered she needed a bachelor's degree for eligibility for the public health credential. At 60, she wasn't sure she wanted to go back to school for the degree that would take 4 or more years, as she could not afford to stop work and attend school full-time. By the time she finished the degree, would she be too old to keep up with that job? She was angry at herself for not planning her career strategy earlier. However, she talked to other nurses and discovered many similarities between her and other nurses her age, several of whom were going to school to prepare for other nursing options.

Some of the most important changes are learned from other professionals who are in positions of influence, such as nurses who serve on hospital committees or from politically active nurses. While we hear a lot about the problems the health care system faces, there are a lot of people out there working to create solutions and change. If you keep close to those who have access to the systems about to change, it is easy to learn about what will occur or not occur. Not only is this knowledge valuable, as it allows nurses to assess their readiness should the change occur, it is also true that opportunities are most prevalent during times of change.

Nurse Practitioner Pioneer

A good example of this need to think ahead and be ready for change is the role nurses play today as nurse practitioners (NPs). There was no such thing as a nurse practitioner before a shortage of physicians in rural Colorado in the 1960s created a health care crisis and prompted a nurse—Loretta Ford—and a physician to develop this role to serve the underserved rural populations. As time passed, that early role developed from a six-week course to a master's degree, with nurses in some areas of the country delivering primary care independent of physicians. Were most nurses ready for that change? No, most were not. In fact, many nurses, as well as physicians, were opposed to the new nurse role. But over time and with support from the nursing associations and the National State Board of Nursing, the role developed so that many nurses today are providing primary care to populations all over the country. Changes such as this one don't occur often, but when they do, nurses need to be ready for the opportunities they provide.

Being ready for change is more than being alert to the changes; it's being prepared for the options that might be available for the change to happen, grow, and flourish. And not all the changes are related to education. Frequently, the changes demand nurses be able to adjust to a new way of delivering care. For example, with advances in technology—the way robotic surgery is performed, for instance, and the way primary care can be delivered by telemedicine—it is clear that nurses must be able to adjust their thinking and their skill sets to meet these new challenges. When the da Vinci system, which is a robotic surgi-

"It is essential nurses know what is expected and be prepared to adjust and adopt new skills."

cal system, is used to perform surgery, the scrub nurse is required to perform very different tasks than were needed when the physicians did the surgery using their own hands. The same can be said about the delivery of primary care via interactive video. The nurse's role is quite different when the care delivery is from the physician's office to the home of the patient via interactive television. And when "ROBODOC" makes rounds, the nurse's role is different than it is when the doctor is standing beside that nurse and talking directly with the patient.

It is not enough to know about these changes. It is essential nurses know what is expected and be prepared to adjust and adopt new skills. This would mean nurses need to do one or all of the following:

- Join a national organization of their specialty

- Return to school and learn more about health care system changes

- Volunteer at a local acute care setting to learn more about what is currently happening in the local area

- Subscribe to a nursing journal related to their specialty

Activity 5: Build Networks

Having a link to someone who is knowledgeable, who has access to opportunities, and who has an influential network is important. Building and maintaining relationships can be time-consuming but almost always pays off in big dividends. Many of these relationships start in school, and others occur during the first few career years. Today, mentoring programs for recent graduates are common, so the linkages can start early. Whether they are school- or work-related, bonds with experienced nurses, physicians, and other health care professionals are

"The development of a network of mentors/helpers is the best way to ensure someone is available to keep nurses informed about the options available and the ways to prepare for them."

excellent ways to learn more about what is happening in the work-place and what is needed.

There is a lot of information out there about the mentoring process and its value as a way to help nurses new to the profession. Less common is information about the value of mentoring Third Age nurses. However, the same issues are experienced by both the new and the older nurse. Having a good role model, someone to discuss an idea with or someone to reflect on an experience with, is just as valuable for the Third Age nurse as it is for the new nurse.

Networks also mean nurses can find "internetwork" help. Nurses can share networks through varying degrees of connections. Those familiar with social networking sites may relate to first, second, and third degree friends or contacts. Another way of looking at the issue is to consider the six degrees of separation principle, whereby everyone is no more than six degrees away from anyone else in the world. It is this direct and indirect networking that often provides nurses with the knowledge and opportunities it takes for the next steps, which are to:

- Locate an old mentor and reconnect with her or him. Have a phone conversation. Write down the potential opportunity seeds this reconnection planted in your mind. Be persistent, but don't persist beyond your comfort level. If you cannot reconnect with one particular person, go to the next one on your list.

- Join an online networking service, such as LinkedIn, which makes it easy to reconnect with a large past network. Go to www.linkedin.com, create a profile, and see how easy it is to have a network of 50 to 100 people just from past jobs.

Being Ready

One nurse told a story about how she had learned so much from her manager about what was going to happen and how she could prepare herself that when the call went out for people interested in the new position, she was ready. She didn't need to return to school or to learn a new skill; she simply had to think about the responsibilities in a new way and to prepare herself to share governance rather than to be the authority when she applied for the position. It was a shift in thinking and in the application of leadership skills from a transactional mode to a transformational mode. She had a good role model and a patient advocate who rehearsed with her and rewarded her when she was able to advocate for and enable others. Without this mentor, she might not have been able to make the needed changes—or have even attempted to change.

Activity 6: Be Flexible

Nurses must be flexible. That is, they must be able to adapt, to change when needed. Whether nurses decide to continue working or retire, the same principles apply. Retirement does not mean doing nothing; if it is to be a rewarding experience, you need to address the same issues in retirement that you would if you continued to work. Without flexibility, nurses will find that neither a new direction in the workplace nor retirement will provide the satisfaction desired.

Flexibility means adaptability, resilience, versatility. While it can mean other things depending on the context, for this purpose it means being able to adjust to new ideas, new expectations, and new roles. It does not mean giving in or giving up one's values or beliefs, but being able to take on new ways of looking at situations and being able to accept them or adjust to a new way of doing something. Flexibility does not mean throwing out everything you know or can do well, but it does mean adjusting your way of seeing and doing things so you are adding to your repertoire, not just dumping the old to make room for the new.

A good example of being flexible is when nurses who have always followed a specific procedure ask themselves, "Why am I doing this?" Being flexible is also evident when the nurse who has always been in control of the situation relinquishes control to the patient, knowing that empowering the patient to make valid, personal decisions is the best way to teach promotion of health. Being flexible also means being ready to work as a team member or the team leader as the situation and the members demand. Knowing when to follow, when to question, and when to alter are all good measurements of flexibility. At times, nurses must adapt even patient protocols for optimum outcomes. The same holds true for careers as it does for patients.

"Frequently, change blocks our ability to see the whole picture. Either we get excited and see only the opportunity and not the challenges, or we see only the barriers and not the opportunities."

While patient protocols are critical and require consistency in most cases, many unique and different Third Age Career roles for nurses do not always lend themselves to step-by-step actions. At times, nurses may be asked to design the action or to alter the activity to fit the needs of the patient, the staff member, or whoever is involved in the experience. At other times nurses are expected to take the lead and help others design the actions to meet a goal.

As health care systems change and more technology becomes commonplace, the need to be flexible means nurses have more opportunities to learn new ways to address the health care needs of the public. Examples of ways to foster and retain a flexible nature are to:

- Practice doing something you love differently, like changing the order in which you complete a task.

- Try a new way to organize your day.

- Arrange your activities so they meet the needs of someone else.

- Seek the advice of another, even when you know what to do.

Activity 7: Develop a Support System

While developing a support system is listed as the last activity in this chapter, it is one of the most important. You could master all of the other six activities, but without support, you will probably not achieve success in the Third Age or in any age. This support could be in the form of a person, people, financial support, or all of the above. We all need to have some kind of backup if things do not work out as planned, some kind of support to keep us on track, or some kind of help when things just do not appear possible. That support is often given by a spouse, a friend, a partner, a teacher, a manager, or another trusted person.

Every new venture pursued, whether planned or accidental, needs the input from the supporter so the nurses can see all of the possibilities, challenges, and potentials. Frequently, change blocks our ability to see the whole picture. Either we get excited and see only the opportunity and not the challenges, or we see only the barriers and not the opportunities. Having another set of eyes helps nurses get the whole picture.

Further, if nurses take the new position or even decide to retire, they need to have someone to talk with about feelings and issues that arise during this critically important point in their lives. Can you remember your first day of nursing school? Besides being excited by the chance to learn something new, were you also frightened by the expectations of the teacher and the demands of the course? It was then that many of us leaned on a roommate for help, someone who was also in the same condition. And in the many instances when the roommate couldn't be of help, we phoned home.

Since support is so critical, it is helpful to try the following:

▪ Establish a nurse support group.

"Having a plan, knowing your strengths and needs, being ready for the future, building networks, being flexible, and having a support system make it easy to answer the question 'What do I want to do next?'"

- Locate a mentor you can trust.

- Create a plan for what you will need if your current support system(s) fails.

- Join an online support group.

- Join a national nurse organization.

Special Challenges

"Having control, preparation, and a sense of your worth and value is important in this pursuit of a career in the Third Age."

After nurses complete these seven activities, the next step is easy because moving forward in career planning really rests on the preparatory activities. Having a plan, knowing your strengths and needs, being ready for the future, building networks, being flexible, and having a support system make it easy to answer the question "What do I want to do next?" The preparatory work defined and explained in this chapter is prerequisite to the process of redirecting your career. And take note: Given this preparation, the question you are more likely to ask yourself is "What can I do given my strengths, needs, and readiness?"

This question and others like it position the path ahead as something designed by nurses and not something merely available. Having control, preparation, and a sense of your worth and value is important in this pursuit of a career in the Third Age.

To get ready for change, you need to consider several other factors and challenges for a successful transition during the Third Age. These transitions usually mean a major change, one that necessitates considerable analysis and thought. Keep in mind, however, that while the issues discussed here are important, they might not be the only ones to consider. Ask yourself, "What behavioral, attitudinal, and physical changes are needed to create a successful experience in my Third Age?"

Going From Inpatient to Outpatient Care

Many nurses love what they are doing, but just cannot keep up with the physical demands of the position. Lifting and other physical patient-care work that was easy at 20, 30, or even 40 may seriously jeopardize your health in your 50s and 60s. At this stage, many nurses think about a position in the community. To do so means a change in more than the physical demands of the job. Community work often demands an attitudinal change.

Hospital nurses are in control of the environment (the hospital room) and the daily activities provided. In the community, the reverse is true. The patient, now known as the client, is in control of the environment, so the approach and expectations of nurses must be different. During a home visit, nurses are visitors, and thus the plan of care is negotiated between the client and the nurse. Assessments are as important in the home as they are in the hospital, but the focus for nurses is now to empower clients to take control of their health and the health of the family (Allender & Spradley, 2005). Promotion of health is the focus, and prevention of illness is the goal, whereas hospital nurses are providing curative inventions. The purpose and goals of community nursing are different.

Many nurses have difficulty with this shift, so before a move from hospital to community is made, Third Age nurses need to learn more about the role of the community health nurse. A course in community health nursing at a college or university is often a good approach, or if nurses have had coursework, a good mentor on the job is helpful. The important thing to remember is the approach is different; thus, nurses must alter their attitudes and expectations accordingly.

Going From Expert to Novice

One of the hardest shifts is to move from the expert in the field to a new learner or novice. It is hard for the expert in one area to accept the novice role in another without feeling "dumb" or "out of place." Many nurses have been reluctant to move into something new, even though they know they cannot stay where they are, because of this fear of looking and feeling inept. We have a few tricks for making this transition easier.

First, nurses need to realize that becoming an expert means they had many things to learn and that the learning occurred all of the time. Thus, learning has always been part of the job. So learning in this new position, different as it might be, is not a new task but something they are very good at. Second, learning something new will probably take less time for experts because they have learned to make change over and over again and thus have learned to do so quickly. Lastly, whereas the focus, expectations, and goals might be different, the expertise gained during the first career always provides nurses with the sense of accomplishment so needed when change occurs. Thus, nurses must always remember and focus on what they have accomplished and use that sense of worth while learning the new role.

> "Learning in this new position, different as it might be, is not a new task but something they are very good at."

Transitioning From Retirement Back to Work

Over and over again, we hear from nurses who have retired and want to return to the workforce. These nurses talk about how hard it is to even get an interview, let alone a job. The first task is to find a good refresher course, one that has a clinical component if hospital work is what is sought. However, a retired nurse can re-enter the workforce in many other ways. Public health nursing, hospice care, occupational nursing, school nursing, parish nursing, visiting nurse care, and many other nonclinical positions are just a few of the opportunities available. The choices are really endless. It just depends on what nurses want to pursue and what requirements must be met.

To determine what is available, start by:

- Searching the Web for jobs

- Locating a return-to-nursing program, whether online or through a local hospital or health care organization

- Joining a professional nursing association

- Going back to school

- Linking up with nurse colleagues

Moving Outside Nursing Care

Moving into something entirely outside of nursing, like a business position or working for design/architectural firms, means the tasks nurses need to accomplish are different. However, nurses must never forget that a nursing education provides nurses with a huge body of knowledge. This body of knowledge provides nurses with valuable information, and when coupled with the years of experience working with people, the transition to another job outside of nursing can be fairly easy. For example, a nurse who had 20 years of experience in bedside care moved to working for a pharmaceutical company, marketing its products to physicians. As a nurse, he knew how to address the concerns of the physicians, what the product could do for the patient, and how the cost/benefit of the product could be addressed.

Another nurse who had several years of experience in maternal/child care went to work for an architectural firm in her hospital design division. Her many years in the hospital gave her the best understanding of what would and would not work when the design of a new or renovated hospital was in process. Furthermore, many nurses have gone to work writing or editing. Years of nursing expertise can be very desirable to anyone publishing nursing periodicals or books.

Moving Into Retirement

Frequently, nurses express an intense desire to retire. While this is clearly an option for many nurses, there are many considerations to factor before quitting a job and leaving the workforce. Ask yourself:

- What can you do that is less demanding but still provides the necessary income?

- What will you do if you leave the workforce that provides you with the satisfaction you need to feel worthwhile and productive?

Many nurses who have quit working have taken up volunteering. For some nurses this work is satisfying. For many others, it is not.

In addition to financial considerations, nurses who are thinking about retirement need to consider three things:

1. How will I use the time?

2. What will help me feel useful?

3. How can I stay connected in case I want to return to work?

Many nurses retire at a point when they are physically and emotionally exhausted. All they can think of is sleeping in and doing all the hobbies and other activities that they put off while work took priority in their lives. One nurse who had been a nurse educator for 30 years decided to retire and do volunteer work. She kept very busy and was satisfied with what she did, but she missed the students. She missed seeing them progress from novices to competent health care providers. She missed being part of their growth. When a call came from a university looking to fill a critical role, she took it and has never regretted returning to work. She learned that time can be filled with useful and productive work, but for her the rewards came from

something that filler activity could not provide her: the personal satisfaction and involvement as a mentor.

References

Allender, J. A., & Spradley, B. W. (2005). *Community health nursing: Promoting and protecting the public's health*. Philadelphia: Lippincott Williams & Wilkins.

Peebles, M. P, (2008). Journey to jobs: Promising paths for nurses. *NurseWeek, 21*(18), 32–33.

Power, S. (2008). Build your bridge: Second careers. Secure path. Retrieved September 5, 2008, from http://www.securepathbytransamerica.com/app/articleBuildYourBridge.htm

Remodeling Retirement and the Workforce III

Redirecting the Career: 5
A Model

When faced with a decision about whether to stay the course, redirect your career, or retire in the traditional way, you face several ways to make the choice. In this chapter, we present a model for helping nurses decide "what's next?" The outcome of that decision usually leads the decision-maker to other decisions—in a domino effect—so the model incorporates several processes nurses can use during their decision-making process.

The model begins with the four K's:

- Know what's needed.

- Know your strengths.

- Know your limitations.

- Know your passions.

Next comes CRAD:

1. _Create_ the life portfolio.

2. _Reflect_ on past career experiences.

3. _Analyze_ the options.

4. _Determine_ the fit.

After you complete the CRAD model, you are ready to prepare for a search by developing a résumé, preparing for an interview, and evaluating the options. This entire process ends with you selecting what to do next. Remember, this is not a linear process. Depending on the decisions you make within the process, you may go back to the various stages within the process. This is not negative. In fact, decision-making demands a back-and-forth process that allows you to reflect, reconsider, and perhaps even change the decision before the entire process is completed. This back and forth helps ensure you are happy with the outcome.

Redirecting Interest (the Four K's)

Know What's Needed

For a complete self-assessment, nurses must know what is needed in the workplace in addition to what their personal and professional needs are. Examples of workplace needs include technological changes, family-centered care initiatives, safe environments, and evidence-based practice, to list but a few. These examples emphasize that nurses must know how to access the research and how to include the family in the plan of care to be up-to-date and useful in an acute care setting. Being current is absolutely essential for nurses. This knowledge is imperative if nurses want to remain in the system, re-enter the system, or change positions within the system no matter in what role.

> "To assess what they need, nurses must know what is needed in the workplace."

For example, knowing what is needed outside the acute care setting is important because care of the public is occurring much more in the community—and in the home—than ever before in history. Length of stay for hospital patients has been reduced with the implementation of managed care to the point that many patients are receiving complicated care delivered by the family and need a nurse to help them through the ordeal.

With the birth of palliative care and hospice, more nurses are needed to help the patients and their families provide a meaningful and painless death either in a hospice agency or in the home. Few nurses even know what the terms *palliative care* and *hospice* mean, let alone the processes and procedures used. So, again, knowing what is happening in health care helps nurses identify opportunities for providing nursing care and what they need to know and do to get involved in this kind of care, turning a potential limitation into a strength.

Know Your Strengths

Nurses who do not know their strengths cannot know what they can offer patients or where they need to strengthen their knowledge or skills. Frequently people are ready to tell themselves what they lack, but it takes more time and effort to identify strengths. In Chapter 4, we discussed how nurses can determine career pathways. Nurses must start this process by knowing what they need in order to move forward or in order to move back into the workplace. (All the activities in Chapter 4 are designed to make this process as complete as possible. Review those activities should you have any questions about determining your personal and professional needs.)

Know Your Limitations

Just as important as knowing your strengths is knowing your limitations. This knowledge is particularly important for Third Age nurses. Age does have its effects, so for many nurses a limitation might be a physical one. For example, many nurses have back problems because of lifting patients, and unfortunately, many are overweight, which can lead to physical problems for them. Others have spent too long in one area and do not know about what occurs elsewhere. For example, many "burned out" nurses have never considered public health nursing or working in a visiting nurse organization where the physical activities are minimal, but cognitive and communication skills are incredibly important. Nor have these nurses thought about working for a pharmaceutical firm, a book publishing company, or an accreditation firm, yet these organizations employ many nurses.

Nurses working in these organizations must have effective communications skills, function as team members and team leaders within multidisciplinary teams, set agency and personal goals, and keep current regarding the focus of the operation. For many nurses, these skills and responsibilities might be limitations, because they are often not expected of hospital nurses who deliver care at the bedside. However, if you desire to make a change, these might be limitations you need to master as competencies. So again, nurses need to know what is expected so limitations can change into strengths.

Know Your Passions

The last "K" to address is knowing what "turns you on"—in other words, what is your passion. Sometimes this can be the excitement of the job. Sometimes it is the reverse, the lack of demand in the role. It can also be the chance to do something new or the opportunity to expand your repertoire of skills. Whatever it is, you should make an effort to determine what your next move should be based on your passions.

To begin, nurses should examine the past, that is, what has been the most important aspect of the past position(s) or the present one and how that can be retained in something new. For example, one nurse had always worked in pediatrics, but she found it was more difficult coping with the stress and demands of the job. So, she started to ask herself what it was in this present position she liked most. She determined it was working with children and knowing that what she did made a difference in their lives. Next, she started to look for a job where she could work with children, have a little more freedom, and feel less physical stress. She considered applying for a school nurse position and a public health nurse position and discovered she would need credentials for both. This fact meant she would have to return to school, and because she did not want to do that at her age, she considered working in a pediatric physician's office. She did her homework and discovered the salary and the benefits were much better for the school nurse or the public health nurse, so she decided to return to school. Currently, she works as a school nurse and has never been happier in a job.

Another way to begin this process is to do an assessment by asking the question "If I could do anything I wanted, what would be the most fun or rewarding?" For some nurses, the answer is the chance to help others, the opportunity to make a difference, or the chance to do something they never considered a possibility. This last point has happened to many nurses. For example, one nurse was terminated several years ago during a "downsizing" of health care operations. She was devastated. However, a friend heard about her dilemma and offered her a job with an architectural firm. She knew she had no chance of finding another position in an acute care setting, so she said yes without really knowing what she would do. Today this nurse is one of the vice presidents of the organization and spends her time traveling all over the world with a team of architects who design new and exciting innovations for hospitals. She has learned much about what is needed in today's health care systems and how to present these ideas to hospital administrators. What turned her on was being part of a team of innovative thinkers, using the knowledge she had acquired during 15 years of acute care work. She loves the chance to make a difference and to be seen as an expert in her field. For her, innovation is her passion and having the opportunity to make a difference is what keeps her motivated and aware of her skills.

> "Over and over again, we hear nurses saying, 'If I had only known more about my options and where they would lead me, I would have done something quite different.'"

Assessing Readiness (CRAD Process)

The next step in the process of making a decision about the future of your career is to pursue the CRAD process. Nurses need to perform this activity to assess their readiness for a change. Whereas many nurses claim they cannot continue as is or are anxious to return to the workplace, many are really not ready because they do not know what they want to do or where they want to be in the next few years. Thus, they need to complete the life portfolio described in Chapter 1.

Creating the Life Portfolio

Why create a life portfolio if you only want to make this one change? This is a good question, and one the life portfolio process can answer. When you pursue the process of looking forward, you need to determine more than just the next step. Over and over again, we hear nurses saying, "If I had only known more about my options and where they would lead me, I would have done something quite different." The life portfolio forces nurses to look beyond tomorrow and to think about the end goal and how each step (or position) gets them to that goal.

For example, one nurse determined at graduation from college with a BSN degree that he ultimately wanted to be the chief nurse administrator in an acute care setting. He knew this goal meant more education and a great deal of experience in a variety of areas of the hospital, so he could gain an overall understanding of how the parts contributed to the whole. He plotted out a set of positions he needed to pursue and a timeline of when he would return to school to obtain his master's degree. During this process, he learned of a university that offered an MSN/MBA dual-degree program that could be completed in 2 years. He registered for the program 2 years later, kept his evening job in the emergency department, and applied for an opening in the hospital for a manager position. He got the job, went to school once a month when classes for the MSN/MBA were offered, and in 2 years graduated with both degrees. He was promoted to the chief nurse executive 1 year later. The last time we checked in on him, he was waiting to find out if he had been selected as the CEO of a hospital in another state. Even if he does not get this position, he is not worried because he knows his education and his effectiveness as a nurse leader are ultimately going to help him obtain the position he set out to obtain.

Reflect on Your Past Career

An important aspect of completing the life portfolio is to examine or reflect on your past career or positions. Was the job rewarding, challenging, interesting, fulfilling, overwhelming, or stressful? Whatever the job, what do you remember the most? If it was rewarding to you, what specifically did that mean? Did it make you feel like you were making a difference? Reflect on the experience and note in writing what exactly made it rewarding. Do the same with those experiences that were stressful. Describe the exact activities or events that made it stressful.

One nurse who took the time to reflect found that even when her back was killing her with pain, she loved the feeling she got when the patient said "thanks." She learned she loved the way she was able to make patients comfortable even though she was very uncomfortable. So, while she loved the ability to help others, the work was just too much for her physically. She left that position and moved to teaching, where she could share with others what she knew worked, yet was not in pain because of the physical stress of the job. She also found it rewarding to know that while she could help others, her students could also do the same. So, her knowledge and skill were multiplied by the number of students she could teach.

"Reflection is also useful for determining what is working and what is not and whether or not you have an opportunity to make a change."

Reflection is also useful for determining what is working and what is not and whether you have an opportunity to make a change. There are two kinds of reflection: on-action and off-action (Johns & Freshwater, 2005). On-action reflection is when one reflects on an action while involved in the action. It is like nurses asking themselves if the medication being given is the correct dosage just before it is administered. Off-action reflection is when nurses reflect on the day's activities when driving home. When you are examining a job, the reflection is off-action, which gives you the opportunity to determine just what about the position was rewarding and what was stressful or not rewarding.

"Reflection provides a way for identifying what is not worth repeating and what should be avoided."

Reflection provides a way for identifying what is not worth repeating and what should be avoided. Many nurses have left one position or agency and moved to another, only to discover the same problems at the new site as at the old one. This situation happens because nurses have not used reflection to determine what they want to avoid, what they want to seek, or how those fit into the future (Chinn, 2008).

Analyze the Options

After you have determined what you want to avoid and what you want your path ahead to be, the next step is to determine what is available and whether it falls within the desired framework. Nurses should search for positions that are available and then analyze the options to determine which to pursue. While this seems like an easy task—and it is—it does take some time and the ability to use a variety of search tools.

Nurses need to search the Web, check the latest editions of the professional literature, check media resources, talk with those who are involved in health care change (such as leaders of professional organizations), and visit some acute and community health care agencies to see what is happening. They can perform much of this search at the computer, but some of it needs to occur outside the home and work-place. It does take time, but it's time well-spent and can help nurses choose the best position for their needs.

During this phase of the decision-making model, nurses have reached the place where they must analyze their options. At this time, nurses need to reflect on the past to help determine which option to select. For example, one nurse found herself at this juncture and reflected, "While I love the fast pace of the emergency department and the variety of patients I see there, I cannot continue at this pace, but I do not want to take a position that is slow and boring." She did her homework and found five positions she thought she might enjoy given her past work experience:

- One was in a community-based clinic for the uninsured.

- One was at a college of nursing where she could teach acute care.

- One was at an acute hospital in a step-down unit.

- One was at a hospital in the nursing education department.

- One was at a nursing association where she would be in charge of the programs related to acute care.

She struggled with the decision because she thought she might do well and feel fulfilled in any of them.

This point is when the last aspect of the decision model comes into the picture. She needed to determine the fit of the position given her experience, what she had learned through reflection was best for her, and what she truly wanted to do.

Determine Your Fit

To determine your "fit," your entire decision-making process comes to the forefront. After you have completed a review of the life portfolio, know whether it is the right time to make a change, and analyzed your options, you can make your decision. You need to ask several questions:

- Does the position fit into the life portfolio, that is, will it get me to the ultimate outcome?

- Is the position right in terms of where I am today on that pathway?

- Is one option more likely to satisfy my needs as a nurse, yet get me to the ultimate goal?

- Most importantly, which of these options is the least stressful? That was the reason for considering a change.

"The 'fit' is a position that leads to the ultimate career goal, is rewarding in terms of physical and psychological comfort, and is free of the issues that have necessitated a change from the current position."

These questions and perhaps others are important as they determine the fit, which is to find a position that leads to the ultimate career goal, is rewarding in terms of physical and psychological comfort, and is free of the issues that have necessitated a change from the current position. In the case of the nurse previously described, she selected the position in the hospital in the nursing education department, because she did not want to leave the acute care setting and knew she would be working with the nurses and staff of the emergency department when she prepared programs for them. It kept her close to what she loved, yet away from the stress of the department and the physical demands of the position. It also allowed her to learn a new skill, which, according to her life portfolio, allowed her to expand her opportunities down the line as she grew older.

Preparing for the Next Steps

After you have made the decision about which direction to take—whether to redirect the career, take retirement, move on to volunteer activities, or even stay with the current job for a while—you need to prepare for the next step by updating your current résumé or by preparing a résumé or a curriculum vita (CV). Even if your decision is to retire, a résumé is needed because you never know when you might want to re-enter the workplace.

Preparing the Résumé

Every person seeking a job needs to have a résumé or CV, because they are a key marketing tool. The purpose of both, according to Donna Cardillo in her 2008 book, *The Ultimate Career Guide for Nurses*, is "to highlight your most interesting, significant, and marketable skills and experiences. It is a synopsis of your credentials, achievements, skill set, and work history. It is a snapshot of your entire career" (p. 89). Some nurses who have been out of the workforce for awhile find it difficult to prepare a résumé or CV, or even to know the difference.

So, the first question is clear: "What is the difference between a résumé and a curriculum vita (CV)?"

Essentially, they are similar but different and are related to the setting and position. However, the CV might be longer because it is used in the academic world and includes more than the person's positions. It includes the person's education, academic committee work, research, awards, publications, consultations, grant activity, and other activities so important in the world of academia. On the other hand, the résumé also includes a history of the nurse's positions, education, and other activities that are related to the discipline. For nurses, this means a review of the following: licenses and certifications, professional affiliations, presentations, volunteer/community services, and special skills. (See figures 5.1 and 5.2 for examples of a CV and a résumé.)

George Smith, RN, PhD

12345 University Boulevard   •   Indianapolis, Indiana, 10101
111.654.7890   •   george.smith@smith.com

EDUCATION

2000	University of Northern California	PhD
1980	University of Northern California	MSN
1970	California State University	BSN

EXPERIENCE—TEACHING

2005–present	Associate Dean, School of Nursing Central State University
1998–2005	Professor, Department of Nursing Midstate University
1994–1998	Associate Professor North Central College
1988–1994	Assistant Professor University of America
1985–1988	Lecturer, School of Nursing Community College

EXPERIENCE—NURSE WORK

1970–1985	Staff Nurse University Hospital

PUBLICATIONS

Smith, G., and Jordan, P. (2004). Using evidence to establish protocols, *Leaders in Nursing, 33*(2), 5–9.

Smith, G. (1990). *Evidence-based practice: Basis for emergency care*. Doctoral Dissertation

PRESENTATIONS

Evidence-Based Practice: Presentation College, Andrews, South Dakota, May 2007

Applying Evidence to Practice: California University, April 2007

Searching the Literature for Evidence: Samson College, Omaha, Nebraska, November 2006

A Career as Faculty: Warden College, San Rafael, California, April 2005

How to Use Evidence in Practice: Unity College, San Bernardino, December 2004

Using Evidence to Improve Leadership Skills: Lutheran University, Washington, DC, November 2003

What is Evidence-Based Practice?: University of South Carolina, Spartanburg, September 2002

How to Begin a Literature Search for Evidence-Based Practice: Ohio University, School of Nursing, Athens, Ohio, October 2001

RESEARCH

Use of Evidence-based Practice on the Effects of Preoperative Instruction of Patients on PCA and Their Ability to Use the PCA to Manage Their Pain, 2005

Effects of Teaching Evidence-based Practice on the Critical Elements of Psychomotor Skills to Baccalaureate Nursing Students, 2000

Administrative Structure of Schools/Departments of Nursing in Private Universities/Colleges, 1995

Perceptions of ADN and BSN Graduates on the Effect of Education of Nurses Related to Job Advancement, 1991

Figure 5.1   Example of a curriculum vita (CV)

Jane Doe

12345 Hospital Boulevard   •   Indianapolis, Indiana, 10101
111.654.7890   •   jane.doe@doe.com

OVERVIEW

Looking for a nursing position in the community where I can offer my skills as an effective communicator and efficient leader with nearly 30 years experience as a staff nurse in acute care facilities, and with an interest in helping the disadvantaged.

EDUCATION

MSN (FNP)	General University (will graduate in May 2009)	2009
BSN	University of Central California	1985
ADN	University of Northern California	1980
Diploma Graduate	Central Hospital	1970

LICENSES/CERTIFICATIONS

Registered Nurse in the State of California

Certified for Advanced Cardiac Life Support (ACLS)

National Certification Exam for Family Nurse Practitioner (after graduation in May 2009)

EXPERIENCE

1990–present   Lawrenceville Medical Center

- Hired as a staff nurse on a general medical-surgical unit
- Promoted to unit manager after the first year so decided to return to school
- Lead manager on the hospital committee to implement evidence-based practice
- Member of a hospital-wide committee to address the incidence of falls
- Led the team that developed the SBAR protocols

1980–1990   Journeyville Community Hospital

- Hired as a staff nurse on a adult-care unit
- Preceptor to nursing students from local colleges
- Member of the committee that developed protocols for patients at-risk during hospitalization
- Led the committee that developed an orientation program for new hires

1970–1980   Watson Hospital

- Hired as a new graduate
- Managed the care of a group of patients as team leader of a group of nurses and nurse aids
- Acted as assistant manager when staffing for the position was difficult
- Helped establish protocols for mediation administration

PROFESSIONAL MEMBERSHIPS

American Nurses Association
California Nurses Association
The Honor Society of Nursing, Sigma Theta Tau International

SPECIAL SKILLS

Can provide sign language for the deaf

Is proficient in a review of the literature when working on evidence-based practice

Is an excellent role model who demonstrates a team approach

SAMPLE AWARDS

Nurse of the Month Award (3 times) over the last 15 years
Received the Best Nurse Preceptor/Mentor Award in 2007

Figure 5.2   Example of a résumé

While you can choose from several formats for the preparation of a résumé or CV, most use chronological order because it begins with the most current work experience, followed by a list of the other positions in reverse chronological format. Each position is listed showing a progressive employment history. The same process is used to list the education, presentations, and the activities listed under each category.

Human resource professionals and hiring managers are accustomed to scanning CVs and résumés for an overview of the applicant's activities and readiness for the position. Here are some basic tips making your CV or résumé make that first cut:

- Use a common 12-point font such as Times New Roman when creating the document. If the font or the size make it difficult to read, it will more than likely be passed over quickly.

- Type in black ink on white paper for readability.

- Avoid pictures, logos, or other images. They distract from the important information.

- Place your name at the top of the page and include your credentials.

- Use 1-inch margins on all 4 sides of the paper.

- Put the categories (education, presentations, etc.) in capital letters. Place them in the center of the page and then list the activities in each category below in chronological order.

- Keep the lists to a 10–15 year history.

- Include all work experiences, even those beyond nursing.

In the résumé, describe what you did in each position. Use bullet points to keep the descriptions short and succinct.

Try to keep the résumé to one or two pages. The CV will be longer.

- Do not type résumé or curriculum vita at the top of the document. Employers know by reading the document what it is.

- The order of the résumé or CV begins with a list of educational experiences and is followed by the work experiences and then by the other categories. This arrangement gives readers an overview of the background preparation for the positions, the list of the positions and what was accomplished, and the other activities that might or might not support the positions.

Preparing the Cover Letter

After the résumé or CV is completed, the next step is to prepare a cover letter. The cover letter, unlike the résumé or CV, should be different for each position. It is a personal approach to get the employer to read your résumé or CV. In the cover letter, you can reveal a bit of your personality and individuality. Highlight specific experiences, credentials, and personal characteristics that relate to the position (Cardillo, 2008).

The cover letter should be organized into three sections:

- An introduction

- The body of the letter

- A summary

In other words, you want to introduce yourself and tell readers where you heard about the position in the introduction. In the body of the letter you want to make the case that you have the qualifications and experiences for the job, and in the summary you want to reiterate why you want readers to review your résumé or CV and invite them to give you a call if they would like an interview.

Also, do not address the letter to "Whom it may concern." If you do not have a name, address the letter to "Dear Recruiter," "Dear Human Resource Manager," or something like that, and end the letter with "Sincerely yours."

Keep the letter to one page, be grammatically correct, and avoid spelling errors. To catch errors, it helps to have someone else review the letter before it is mailed. As with the CV or résumé, make sure the letter is on white paper with black type; it should never be handwritten. The cover letter can be mailed or placed on the Web. It is not a good idea to fax it, because you never know if the person you want to get it ever sees it or if it arrives in the best condition. If you have a business card, include it with the cover letter and résumé or CV when they are mailed.

Getting Ready for the Interview

Just showing up for an interview is not enough, regardless of whether there is a shortage of nurses or not. Employers are paying a high price for the frequent "turnover" rates of nurses, as 40,000 new nurses leave the workplace each year after only 1 year of employment (Shapiro & Krause, 2008). Employers have become very careful when hiring new personnel, which means nurses must be prepared for the interview. For some, the interview is an anxiety-provoking experience, particularly if it has been awhile since their most recent interview.

> "Employers are paying a high price for the frequent 'turnover' rates of nurses, so they have become very careful when hiring new personnel."

The interview is an opportunity for both interviewers and nurses to obtain more information. For interviewers, it is an opportunity to determine if a nurse is the right person for the position. For nurses it is an opportunity to present themselves in the best way possible and to learn more about the position and if the fit is right after all.

Thus, nurses need to pose several questions to learn more about the position, while also making the best effort possible to convince the interviewer they are right for the position. Start with finding out who is conducting the interview and where the interview is going to take place. After these are known, nurses need to consider the following:

- What to wear. Always err on the side of professional attire unless instructed otherwise.

- What to bring. Always bring extra résumés or CVs—as sometimes you will be invited to interview with other personnel on the spot to expedite the process—and a notebook for taking notes.

- How to address the interviewer. Ideally, get his or her credentials so you can know whether to use "doctor."

- What to say at the beginning of the interview. For example, introduce yourself and tell why you are interested in the position. Sitting quietly may send the wrong message.

- Questions to ask about the position. For example, why is the position open? This helps you get an idea of the turnover rate.

Ask your contacts, those who know the institution before the interview, to learn more about the work environment and if workers are supported. In this way you can also learn more about management style and if problems recur in this area.

Interviews are a two-way street. While the major reason for the interview is for nurses to make the best impression and convince the interviewer they are right for the position, it is important that nurses get as much information during the interview as they need to make an informed decision for themselves. Consider asking the following questions to learn as much as possible about expectations and employee support:

- Is there an orientation program?

- What are the challenges of the position?

- What are the opportunities of the position?

- What are the working hours? Is overtime required?

- How is staffing determined?

- What are you looking for in this new employee?

- What kind of previous experience do you prefer?

- When will the position to be filled?

- Can I talk with a staff member?

While these questions are important and need answers, it's also important to time your questions to the appropriate place in the interview. Common sense is the best judge of timing, as it is with any conversation. For instance, asking when the position will be filled should be one of the last questions—as the interview is wrapping up, never at the beginning. Do not fire your questions at the interviewer all at once.

A major aspect of the interview is making positive eye contact and developing good rapport. The first part of the interview should be in the hands of the interviewer. While answering questions, be aware that nonverbal communication is very important. Body position, facial expressions, and the words chosen are significant. The best advice is to remain calm, answer the questions using short but complete sentences, and avoid saying anything negative about past employers.

If you are asked, "Why are you considering leaving your current job?" or "Why is there a 5-year gap in your résumé?," be honest and take responsibility for the reasons. This is the juncture of the interview where the reasons for a return to the workforce or a change are related to the opportunity this particular position offers; discussing that says something about your understanding of the importance of the position and provides you with an opportunity to share your expertise and make clear that you have the qualities they are seeking.

In many instances, interviewers may simply turn to interviewees and ask them why they think they are appropriate for the position. Nurses can then elaborate on their skills and qualities. Why do they want the job? Why do they want to work for this particular company? How does this position fit into their career? At this time nurses can provide a full disclosure of their talents.

When it appears an interviewer is completing his or her questions, nurses can then ask three final questions:

- Is there anything else I need to tell you?

- When can I expect to hear from you about whether I am being considered for the position?

- Are there others being considered for the position?

These questions allow nurses to know if interviewers have any questions about their qualifications or skills and past history and if they have hope of getting the job. Leaving an interview without this information might mean nurses walk away with a distorted view of the outcome; the reality might be much different than they perceive.

Every interview is different, and every interview provides nurses with new knowledge about how to improve. Many nurses leave an interview with high hopes only to find out later the job went to someone else, and they never know why. Third Age nurses are not novices in nursing, but they might be novices when it comes to job interviews. Their fear of rejection might be higher than it is for other nurses; however, their chances of obtaining the position are probably better than most, even if they are re-entering the workforce, because of their years of experience. And though the experience might be different and not necessarily related to the job they are interviewing for, their maturity is always a plus.

Employers are looking for responsible and reliable workers, and older nurses are known for these qualities. They are also known for their ability to quickly learn new ways to provide care, even if they are in a nonacute care setting and their experience has always been in an acute setting. They can assess patients, make diagnoses, and plan care whether they are in an acute setting or in the community. Also, nurses with advanced degrees are known for their flexibility and eagerness to learn and implement new technologies.

> "Employers are looking for responsible and reliable workers, and older nurses are known for these qualities."

Evaluating the Options

As you evaluate your options, these five questions are crucial to determining next steps:

1. What do you want?

2. What can you offer?

3. Is there anything you need to do to meet the job requirements?

4. Do you want to do the work to meet the job requirements?

5. Is your perfect job out there?

What Do You Want?

The first step in evaluating your options for the future is to go back and review what you want. Is it a new position? Is it trying out an official retirement? Or is it to rest for a while before re-entering the workforce?

If it's a rest you need, then maybe now is not the time to consider a different job or retirement but to take time for that rest. Many nurses have left the workforce to "find" themselves, and many did so through volunteer work with religious or community organizations. As a result, they learned about the many opportunities—with pay—available for nurses. It does not hurt to take the time to review the four K's as a way to evaluate what you have learned about your options.

What Can You Offer?

The next aspect of evaluating options is to determine what it is you are willing to offer or give up if the option is attractive. Too often, nurses are offered a fantastic salary only to discover that the job is ill defined, the resources are limited, or the workplace is hostile. At this juncture, you need to look at all that is needed to succeed, even if the goal is to retire, and what you need to provide to make it a successful experience. Many nurses are so worn out from their present position or situation that they think retirement will solve all their problems and satisfy them. However, many jump into retirement and then find out it doesn't meet their needs. Ask yourself, "If I do not have a job, what will I do with my time?" Again, consider what it takes to make life rewarding and satisfying for you, and then plan and pursue that path.

Is There Anything You Need to Do to Meet the Job Requirements?

Many, especially those interested in remaining in the workforce or getting back into the workforce, need skills to place them in a competitive position for the opportunities available. These skills sometimes require additional education, and sometimes they are ways to retool. For example, frequently when nurses are "burnt out" from the demands of the acute care setting, they start to think about teaching. Unfortunately, because of a lack of the appropriate level of education, many nurses are not properly prepared for a faculty position or even for working in the education department. Going back to school to earn a degree might be the only way nurses can become eligible for the position.

Or, nurses might have been out of the workforce for many years and now want to re-enter, only to find they have to meet many difficult requirements to return. For example, to re-enter the workforce in acute care, nurses must complete a re-entry program that has a clinical aspect. Unfortunately, very few programs of this nature exist, so nurses are unable to return in many cases.

Another good way to begin is to check the Web for what is available, to talk with employed nurses who can ask their human resources person for a referral, or to read the many nurse career journals or blogs that are out there. Almost every professional nurse organization offers continuing education courses—many online—that can help prepare nurses to change or resume a position.

Do You Want to Do the Work to Meet the Job Requirements?

This leads to the next question, "Are the requirements for the job/position what you want to do?" Are you willing and able to go back to school in your later years? Many nurses in their 50s and 60s are seeking a degree. Some are doing well, and some are struggling because their most recent school experience was a long time ago and without the needed support, both at school and home, the experience is not positive. Even a refresher course can be difficult if no support or rewards are gained from the experience.

It is in this area that many nurses are stopped. So the choice of what to do might rest on the desire, fortitude, and stamina of nurses when faced with something as difficult as returning to school when support is minimal and the tasks are difficult.

These barriers clearly make it necessary for nurses who want to make the best choice to assess their own strengths and the support systems available. How much nurses are willing to meet the requirements, given the amount of stress those requirements may create and how much help they have to address the stress, may factor heavily in the decision.

Is Your Perfect Job Out There?

Pretend for a minute that the requirements for the next aspect of your life are not an obstacle and all of the options for a new position or retirement are attractive. The next question to ask is, "Are the options (whatever they are) a fit, given what I think I want and what it will take to become eligible?" This question might take different forms in different situations:

- "Do I really want to go back to school and become a faculty person, given the length of time it takes to get prepared and my desire to teach?"

- "Is teaching going to give me the rewards I am looking for?"

- "Though I am tired now, do I really want to rest for a year or so while I figure out what I want to do?"

- "Is resting what I really want to do?"

- "Are these options a fit for me at this time in my life?"

- "If they do not fit, what is available that is a better fit?"

However, the primary question is this: What does *fit* mean? In this case, it means the outcome of the decision—staying on the job, selecting a new position, or retiring—meets the desires of the decision-maker. For example, are the choices what the decision-maker wants?

Or, do the choices demand something the decision-maker is willing to do to become eligible? Are these demands something the decision-maker is able to accomplish or provide? If the answers to these questions are "yes," then it appears you have a fit. The next step is to select the best fit.

Making the Selection

It is common for people to have more than one option to consider when faced with late-in-life career decisions. For nurses, this point is important because many hospitals and other health care facilities are making the working environment more attractive. For example, Scripps Health in San Diego, California, has been honored nationally as one of the 50 Best Employers for Workers over 50 by AARP for several years in a row (Hatcher, et al., 2006). Ranked number four in the nation in 2007, Scripps is the only San Diego employer and the highest-ranked California employer on the current list. Scripps was recognized for offering benefits that address the various cycles of an employee's life, including phased retirement and flexible scheduling. In 2006, AARP also honored Scripps with its Bernard E. Nash Award for Innovation for a training program offered to Scripps' senior workforce.

Johns Hopkins Medical Center has also been among the hospitals offering programs and opportunities to nurses over 50 that better meet their needs and desires (Shapiro, & Krause, 2008). According to the AARP (2007), 22 hospitals throughout the United States were cited as the "Best Employers for Workers Over 50." Chapter 6 provides a thorough discussion of the opportunities and changes occurring in U.S. hospitals to address the over-50 population of nurses. Be clear that opportunities are available and expanding, so nurses need to know what they want, what is available, and if they have a fit. Thus, the next task is to have a way to make the selection.

The Best Fit

Obviously your choice is made and determined by which option is the best fit. For example, which option meets the desired outcome with the least demands? Which option takes the least amount of change or preparation for the decision-maker? And which option has the greatest potential for the future? However, more than one option may meet the criteria. If this occurs, several other issues can determine the final choice. Is the option close to home, or will a move be needed? Does the best fit mean the decision-maker will need to spend considerable time and money preparing for the position?

Chapter 6 provides a discussion of the changes in health care directed toward older nurses and how various hospitals and health care agencies are changing to address this particular population.

While more new nurses are entering the workforce, a critical shortage remains, and that shortage is not only in numbers but in the loss of experienced and skillful nurses. Much is being spent in money and effort to orient and help the new nurse with entry into the system, but it takes years to develop skill and become a productive, efficient care provider. We really need to address this nurse shortage from two perspectives: with new nurses and with retention of some nurses at or nearing retirement age.

References

AARP. (2007). Best Employers for workers over 50. Retrieved September 15, 2008, from www.aarp.org/bestemployer.

Cardillo, D. W. (2008). *The ultimate career guide for nurses*. Falls Church, VA: Gannett Healthcare Group.

Chinn, P. L. (2008). Reflections on retirement and related matters. In M. H. Ottermann. *Annual Review of Nursing Education*. (pp. 255–269). New York: Springer.

Hatcher, B., Bleich, M. R., Connolly, C., Davis, K., O'Neill, H., & Hill, K. S. (2006). (Eds.) *Wisdom at work: The importance of the older and experienced nurse in the workplace*. Princeton, NJ: Robert Wood Johnson Foundation.

Johns, C., & Freshwater, D. (2005). *Transforming nursing through reflective practice* (2nd edition). Malden, MA: Blackwell.

Shapiro, S., & Krause, J. (2008). Solving the shortage: How can we keep nurses from disappearing? *Johns Hopkins Nursing, VI*(II), 27–33.

Retaining Senior Nurses | **6**

Like many organizations, hospitals are facing formidable crises because of an aging workforce. One crisis that is particularly challenging for hospitals stems from the shortage of nurses. It is predicted that by 2010, 49% of nurses will be older than 50; in 10 more years, 80% of them could be retired if the current pattern of nurses taking retirement at 55 continues (Robert Wood Johnson, 2008). One promising approach to this crisis is to retain senior nurses past retirement age. Throughout this book, we have suggested that nurses can and should rethink and redesign the second half of their lives by using Third Age Life Planning, building Third Age Life/Work Portfolios, and redefining retirement. However, in most cases, nurses cannot move ahead effectively without institutional assistance.

Thus, health care organizations also need to change in order to support the professional growth, personal renewal, and retirement planning of nurses. A panel of experts has affirmed that "nothing short of transformational change is required to avert a potential public health catastrophe within the next 15 years" (Hatcher et al., 2006, p. 53). This transformation calls for creative strategic planning to address the needs of older nurses, to promote their retention, and to improve the quality of patient care.

Why focus on senior nurses? There are two main reasons.

1. Senior nurses are needed to address the projected nurse shortage.

2. They are essential to maintain effective functioning of hospitals.

Third Age nurses know the systems and the best way to care for patients. Because of their experience, knowledge, wisdom, and competence, they provide an invaluable resource. "Nurses are really what people come to hospitals for," remarked a recently retired hospital CEO and Washington-based health care consultant in an interview. Leading professionals who have examined the current crisis have issued this mandate: "The health care industry must aggressively implement workforce strategies to retain nurses as critical knowledge resources and to reduce the cost of turnover" (Hatcher et al., 2006, p. 5). How they might accomplish this mandate is the subject of this chapter.

A few hospital administrators are already ahead of the curve, having initiated organizational transformation several years ago. Some others have initiated innovative strategies, policies, and practices that are promoting senior nurses and implementing strategies aimed at retaining them. This chapter contains suggestions about critical areas to consider for effective change and provides examples to illustrate how hospital administrators can address the issues of an aging workforce and the critical shortage of nurses.

Retention of nurses is a complicated process, requiring many different solutions. There is no one right way to do this. In fact, hospital administrators must develop multiple approaches, ones that are most appropriate to their own unique qualities and situations. However, we have found 12 components that hospital administrators and nurses should consider, and we discuss how a few hospital administrators have responded in specific areas.

An abundance of recent resources inform the construction of this chapter. AARP now has an annual list of Best Employers for Workers Over 50. This list includes detailed reports on nearly two dozen hospitals that have given us a base to work with. Several other publications provide additional information. For example, *Fortune* magazine's 100 Best Companies to Work For in 2008 has selected Scripps Health in San Diego, California. Mercy Health System in Janesville, Wisconsin, was a 2007 recipient of the Malcolm Baldridge National Quality Award. *Working Mother* magazine's Best Companies list includes several hospitals that have cultural changes supporting the development and satisfaction of all nurses. In August 2008, *U.S. News & World Report* provided information on select hospitals regarding the best 19 in the United States. These reports have provided additional information about and insights into outstanding, innovative hospitals. The American Hospital Association's (AHA) *Hospital and Health Networks* magazine, a variety of online reports from the Robert Wood Johnson Foundation—especially *Wisdom at Work* and *Charting Nursing's Future*—and the American Nurses Association's *Online Journal of Issues in Nursing* have also provided helpful data and analyses. Finally, we have learned much from interviews, using onsite visits, e-mail communications, and telephone calls to health care leaders. All of these resources testify to the spirit, creativity, resilience, and leadership that are emerging to meet the nurse/hospital crisis. They show not only how nurses can be retained, but also how health care delivery can be significantly improved.

Laying the Groundwork for Leading Change

The place to start is for hospital administrators to conduct an assessment of their own workforce and their projected needs in the next 10 to 20 years. For example, how many full-time nurses are older than

50? Some hospital administrators have found that more than a third, and sometimes even half, of their nurses are older than 50. These hospitals need to assess what needs to be done to keep the hospital operating effectively in order to sustain quality patient care.

The executives of Scripps Health started designing their approach once they identified that more than one-third of their nurses were already older than 50. Their projections indicated that by 2012, 40% would be 50 and older. The leaders began asking, "How can we create the most attractive work environment to support and retain our valuable employees?" Their responses to this question, and the answers coming from employee surveys, have led to impressive organizational change during the past several years. Reports from many hospitals on AARP's list of Best Employers of Workers Over 50 indicate these hospitals have developed programs in response to employee surveys, interviews, and individual/team suggestions and recommendations.

In addition to local information, administrators can learn from general sources. For example, focused interviews by the Center for Third Age Nurses and many of the national reports already referenced have indicated what many senior nurses don't like about their jobs and why they are considering leaving. Because most have indicated they might be willing to remain working in health care (fewer than 20% are thinking about doing something else), their concerns need to be seriously considered.

What would these nurses change in order to stay in health care?

- **Workload concerns.** Workload concerns are generally at the top of this list. These concerns include physical demands, heavy lifting, constant walking, exhaustion, excessive record-keeping, and extra duties that take them away from direct patient care.

- **Management.** Some nurses report dissatisfaction with their work because of a poor relationship with supervisors and administrators and/or because they feel underappreciated, disrespected, powerless, locked into a bureaucratic system, and underpaid.

- **Work hours.** Many dislike the long shifts and rigid scheduling.

- **Career concerns.** Many identified the lack of opportunities for learning, for developing new skills, and for building fulfilling career paths as an issue.

The above surveys also indicate nurses are more likely to remain if they:

- Have economic incentives.

- Have a supportive work environment with fewer physical demands.

- Are assisted by technology and better ergonomic designs.

- Have good social interactions with peers, physicians, and administrators.

- Have more control over their time and responsibilities and have recognition and respect.

- Are given more opportunities for learning, renewal, and personal development.

- Can try new roles and share in decision-making.

- Receive assistance in planning a transition into retirement, which will make working longer more attractive.

These aspirations of nurses older than 50 are consistent with findings about the life cycle after 50, Third Age Life Planning discussed in

Chapter 1, and retirement management discussed in Chapter 2. To find out what will most likely keep your Third Age hospital nurses in the system, start by asking them.

In developing change strategies, hospital administrators can also be guided by the expertise of business professionals such as Harvard professor John Kotter. From years of experience studying and working with many leading companies, Kotter realized the most successful have in common an eight-stage approach to the change process (1996). The first step is to create a sense of urgency; nothing can kill the intention to lead change more decisively than a sense of complacency and/or wishful thinking that last year's efforts will inevitably lead to next year's success.

A second essential factor is to build the right coalition of people to lead the change. It is critical for all parties—hospital executives, managers, nurses, financial and HR administrators, IT and technical staff, and nurse unions—to communicate openly and to work together in a partnership. Leaders in tune with others in their coalition must develop and communicate a clear, convincing vision and a strategy that allows people to see where the organization is heading, where they fit into the plan, and how everyone can collaborate to move toward that ideal. With a compelling vision that inspires people, such leaders remove obstacles by empowering their people to achieve both individual and organizational goals. They should also reinforce the long-term visionary goals by short-term wins, maintain a spirit of innovation, and anchor changes in the culture. Leading change effectively inspires people to give their best and to stay aboard.

> "Leading change effectively inspires people to give their best and to stay aboard."

These practical lessons from the experience of leading change are reflected in hospitals where administrators have been improving how they treat their employees, especially those who are also responsible for patient care. Executives in top hospitals have led their people to build places that support, reward, develop, and renew nurses and other employees in the pursuit of excellence. If not at first, eventually CEOs will have to lead the change, as Kotter suggests. However, significant change can begin at lower levels, with nurse managers and even clinical nurses rallying forces and experimenting with new behaviors and organizational changes.

Innovative ideas in successful organizations flow both up and down, and in some cases change has been prompted by external forces. For example, New York's new program on public reporting provides a report card on patient satisfaction. With greater public awareness, Mount Sinai Hospital in New York City has begun to formulate new initiatives for nurses to improve the quality of patient care, such as developments in safe patient handling and creation of new positions for senior nurses in the patient discharge process. Even though many hospitals leading change do not have unions, unions can and should join and help foster change efforts.

"Innovative ideas in successful organizations flow both up and down."

Another example of change prompted by external forces is the New York State Nursing Association. This professional organization, which has a strong commitment to senior nurses, has a very positive relationship with Mount Sinai nurse executives who collaborated to design new roles for nurses that challenge, support, and retain them. Whereas most of their nurses are in their 30s, more nurses older than 50 continue working; 6% are older than 60, and a few are older than 70. Examples from leading hospitals and others demonstrate that vital collaboration within a broad coalition contributes to effective operation, heightened morale, improved retention of nurses, better patient care, and even lower costs.

12 Strategic Areas for Nurse Retention

Investigation into the possibility of retaining senior nurses shows the key areas influencing their decisions include compensation, benefits, work satisfaction, opportunities for growth and renewal, health, and their attitude toward retirement. We have identified 12 strategic areas that demonstrate how some innovative hospital administrators have been working with senior nurses to make change.

1. Compensation and Benefits

While not always the most decisive influence in a nurse's decision to remain in the workforce, economic concerns are extremely important and are being addressed by hospital administrators, who have significantly reduced their rate of turnover. Scripps Health, the seventh-largest employer in San Diego County, California, with more than 11,500 employees, has in the past few years made a concerted effort to address the challenges of the nurse shortage with a complex strategy. Its goal was to develop the most attractive work situation possible, measured in part by a "Great Place to Work" survey. In an effort to improve employee satisfaction, retention, and recruitment, Scripps Health executives have a wide-ranging array of initiatives, including special benefits and a competitive salary scale, which have been recognized with numerous awards. Scripps Health has been recognized as a "Best Employer to Work for" by *Fortune* magazine, AARP, *Working Mother* magazine, and as the best employer in San Diego in 2006. These awards applaud Scripps Health's compensation, benefits, leadership development, and employee support programs. Scripps Health now has biannual marketplace salary adjustments, as well as bonuses for employees who meet performance objectives. It also has a full package of health benefits for individuals and their families. To assist employees with long-term financial planning, they are encouraged to invest in a 401(a), for which they receive matching funds. Employees with more than 15 years of service receive 5%; those with more than 20 years of service receive 6% matching funds. These changes help to retain senior nurses, 40% of whom will be older than 50 in a few years.

Mercy Health System in southern Wisconsin has been recognized by the Malcolm Baldridge National Quality Award for a variety of innovations that support employees' performance and development. Compensation and benefits have not been ignored. The CEO of Mercy Health System has commented, "If you put the effort in up front, it is worth it. We have kept people we would have lost in their early 50s" (*Hospital & Health Networks,* 2008, p. 2.) Already more than 30% of the nurses at Mercy Health System are older than 50, and the turnover rate has dropped from 13.5% to 7%. Employees receive a full benefit package with individual and family insurance for prescriptions, drugs, dental, vision, and long-term care. Mercy Health System administrators also encourage nurses to invest in a 403(b) plan with matching funds. Employees older than 50 can make catch-up contributions to build their pension reserve. They also have paid time off for caregiving—seniors are allowed up to 360 hours.

Many of the hospitals listed in AARP's 2007 Best Employers for Workers over 50 have similar benefit packages, with some allowing full benefits to those working at least 20 to 30 hours a week. Such possibilities encourage nurses to remain, even while cutting down on the number of hours they work. Many reported the improvements in benefits were made in response to employee surveys. For example, St. John Health in Warren, Michigan, eliminated a 35-year maximum service accrual for a defined benefits pension plan and expanded a full health care package for individuals and their families to both full-time and part-time nurses working at least 20 hours a week. Centegra Health System in Woodstock, Illinois, increased the benefit package as well, adding short-term disability insurance for full-time employees and assistance with out-of-pocket health care costs. Rush-Copley Medical Center in Aurora, Illinois, similarly responded to employee surveys with enhanced benefits for health care, adding free memberships to sports facilities and emergency paid time off. The best employers value their nurses, compensate

"The best employers value their nurses, compensate them well, and are responsive to their needs and requests by designing supportive benefit packages."

them well, and are responsive to their needs and requests by designing supportive benefit packages.

2. Workload and Schedules

Almost all hospitals ranked by AARP's 2007 Best Employers for Workers Over 50 have responded to senior nurses' frustrations, needs, and desires with respect to the time requirements of their jobs. Some of the largest, most prestigious hospitals have a wide variety of options, but smaller, less well-known hospitals have also made a concerted effort to retain senior nurses by allowing them to redesign their work schedules. Nurses working at Mercy Health System have many choices, including flexible schedules of 8-, 10-, and 12-hour shifts for full- and part-time nurses, weekend-only shifts, self-designed traveler and floating options, and ways to reduce time at work in phased retirement. Employees older than 55 with 15 years of service can reduce hours and even work at home when possible. At Yale-New Haven Hospital in New Haven, Connecticut, senior nurses enjoy a "Have it Your Way" program that allows fewer hours and flexible scheduling. At Massachusetts General Hospital in Boston, Massachusetts, senior nurses have many options, with flex schedules, weekends only, 4- to 6-hour shifts, self-scheduling, rotating work, and a phased retirement program with part-time work. Senior nurses at Scripps Health have access to a Life Cycle Employment Program, which is specifically designed to provide flexible options, including flex time, compressed work schedules, job sharing, and a phased retirement program that allows full-time nurses to move to part-time status with full benefits and their pension plan intact. Changes in the workload such as these we have mentioned are in sync with the changing expectations, needs, and aspirations of Third Age individuals discussed in Chapter 1.

Smaller, less well-known hospitals also have programs that provide senior nurses with alternative work arrangements, enabling them to downshift time on the job as they approach retirement. Most of these allow full-time nurses to have more free personal time, moving to part-time status while retaining full benefits and pension plans. Rush-Copley Medical Center has an arrangement where senior nurses can move into part-time on either a permanent or temporary basis. Centegra Health System's nurses can choose 10- or 12-hour shifts, weekends only, and part-time status with summers off. Scottsdale Healthcare in Scottsdale, Arizona, has a "Seasonal Leave Program" for senior nurses who are approaching retirement but are not yet ready for full retirement. In addition to reducing hours, senior nurses can also work just 6 months and take a 6-month leave with full benefits paid by the employer. This in effect gives them a sabbatical to experience renewal and have the opportunity for concentrated Third Age Life Planning. Saint Barnabas in West Orange, New Jersey, in addition to flex time for senior nurses, has a per diem nurse program with 1,500 RNs, 320 of whom are older than 50. These nurses receive premium pay in lieu of benefits. West Virginia University Hospital in Morgantown, West Virginia, also includes a per diem option, as well as multiple incentives for senior nurses to remain working toward retirement with reduced hours, flexible schedules, weekends only, and job sharing when possible. Nurses working 20 hours per week can retain full benefits and participation in a 403(b) plan. Like those of some leading corporate enterprises, the administrators of these hospitals have developed ways to keep the professionals they can't really afford to lose by working with them to redesign how and when they work.

3. Workload and Ergonomics

A frequent complaint of senior nurses is exhaustion from physical demands, such as heavy lifting, too much walking, and work-related stress factors. The American Nurses Association's (ANA) *Online Journal of Issues in Nursing* has reported that nurses suffer a disproportionate amount of musculoskeletal disorders because of repeated patient handling (Castro, 2004). Some leading hospital CEOs have recognized the need to reassess how the work environment is designed, as well as how new technology can be used to assist in patient care.

The Greenville Hospital System University Medical Center in Greenville, South Carolina, is an example of how new technology and ergonomics can be used to provide an effective way to correct a dangerous situation for the benefit of both nurses and patients. In 2002, nurse leaders realized they would be facing a critical shortage of nurses in the near future. They began a recruiting process to hire 500 new nurses, and they asked the question, "How can we retain our senior nurses?" Because 36% of their nurses were older than 50, that question needed some good answers. To improve the work environment, they improved compensation and the flow of communication. Feedback from nurses led them to focus on the work environment as an effective way to retain senior nurses and to promote safe patient handling. Like other hospitals where evidence-based practice was used, new lifting technology was introduced into the hospital. It made a huge difference in alleviating handling stress by helping nurses move and transfer patients, which reduced injuries. The technology was introduced into all five of its hospitals with help from a Robert Wood Johnson Foundation grant in 2007.

Like other leading hospitals that have implemented Planetree, the focus here was on ergonomic issues, especially those affecting nurses. The hospital environment was modified with improvements such as:

- Softer flooring for nurses to walk on

- Self-propelled patient beds that are easier to move

- Mini-stations instead of central stations, allowing nurses to observe their patients without having to walk down long corridors to patient rooms

■ Supply cabinets located near patients' rooms

■ A nurse-ergonomist position to focus on patient handling

*Planetree, a nonprofit located in Derby, Connecticut, promotes the development and implementation of innovative models of health care that focus on healing and nurturing body, mind, and spirit.

By listening to nurses' concerns and suggestions, leaders at Green-ville Hospital System University Medical Center have been able to keep their experienced and older skilled nurses and to improve patient care while doing so.

4. Shared Governance

Top organizations in most industries have been moving away from top-down, command-and-control leaders and managers to shared governance that empowers employees to collaboratively achieve both individual and corporate goals. Senior nurses have expressed a strong interest in empowerment and in achieving heightened professional status with more autonomy, trust, shared decision making, leadership development, and recognition. Enlightened hospital administrators have recognized that to retain these nurses, they have to change the way they govern. For example, in the past several years Yale-New Haven Hospital has developed a distinctive form of shared gover-nance. Top leaders have been shaping a culture of collaboration. They promote leadership development, especially of mature nurses, making it an employer of choice. Nurses are involved throughout the insti-tution in shaping the culture and making decisions that affect them and patient care. After a tradition of top-down nursing management, nurse leaders shaped a new governance model; it has begun partnering with its 2,000-menber nursing staff. A first step was to create a Nurse Cabinet made up of all nurse directors, who meet regularly with a new, important body—The Staff Nurse Council—composed of elected nurses. This Council ensures clinical nurses have a significant role in decisions and policy making. With these bodies in place, nurses' ideas, questions, and solutions to problems are communicated broadly as part of hospital leadership.

In addition to previously mentioned innovations, Scripps Health has deliberately created an empowered workforce, particularly through its outstanding leadership development programs, which are part of its commitment to retain experienced, senior nurses. Empowerment is too often an empty term, applied without consideration of what people need to operate more autonomously and effectively. In addition to requisite resources, empowered employees need education and help developing what they learn. Scripps Health has a Center for Learning where employees receive education and develop new skills to move into positions of greater responsibility. One hundred percent of its workforce participated in this program with an average of at least 20 hours. It was particularly relevant to senior nurses who want to improve their leadership status. Nurses can also participate in a "build talent" program within the new Talent Development Center. They receive professional and financial support to advance their careers into higher paying clinical and leadership positions. They have a strong shared governance system of empowered teams and dynamic collaboration. According to one nurse leader, "I can't imagine how any hospital can function without it."

Other hospitals have shared governance that involves senior nurses in specific areas, such as the quality of the work environment and patient care in the Greenville Hospital System. Rush-Copley Medical Center is giving nurses more control over patient flow, admission, and discharge. Most hospitals in the AARP list have strategies, policies, and practices that were changed in response to input from employees. New governance strategies include

1. Developing nurses older than 50 instead of directing them toward retirement pastures outside the walls.

2. Giving them greater voice in decisions instead of expecting silent compliance.

3. Building partnerships among nurses, physicians, administrators, and staff.

4. Recognizing these nurses' knowledge, wisdom, and experience as key.

These can go a long way to keeping senior nurses in the system, adding value to patient care and hospital operations.

Mercy Health System, which in 20 years has grown from a single community hospital to a complex organization with three hospitals and more than 50 outside clinics in Southern Wisconsin and Northern Illinois, has a redefined definition of employees. Rather than calling them *employees*, they call them *partners*. While shared governance has not yet been developed, the institutional philosophy implies engaged, empowered, and valued partners are vital to exceptional health care practices. Partners, especially nurses and physicians, are committed to achieving the Mercy Health System mission of care where patients come first. Partners participate in performance improvement efforts, treat each other like family, and create personal and professional growth and development plans. Further, at Mercy Health System informal methods to bolster empowerment, such as CEO partner forums and lunches with leaders, are in place. As a result, 96% of employees report "feeling valued" and "satisfied." Staff turnover has declined significantly. AARP has ranked Mercy Health System first or second in its Best Employers for Workers Over 50 for several years. In 2007, Mercy Health System won the Malcolm Baldridge National Quality Award. Senior nurses who feel valued and have a say about how things go at work are more inclined to remain there.

"Rather than calling them *employees,* they call them *partners.*"

5. New Roles for Senior Nurses

When asked if they would consider remaining in health care after retirement age, most nurses said they would if they could change how they "nurse." A major component in a change strategy is to invent new roles for nurses that allow them to have the work that suits their stage of development and provides valuable service to the hospital and patient care. Marcia Canton, PhD, RN, who conducted many focused interviews for the Center for Third Age Nurses, sees several such possibilities:

> "When asked if they would consider remaining in health care after retirement age, most nurses said they would if they could change how they 'nurse.'"

Third Age nurses could serve as mentors to teach and support new nurses, and also serve as role models. They could contribute to research and development of nursing, combining traditional skills with the new focus on evidence-based practice. They can also serve as preceptors to assist new graduates in translating theory into practice. (Personal communication with Marcia Canton on September 12, 2008.)

Many senior nurses have said that with all their experience and knowledge, they have a strong desire to impart their wisdom to younger nurses as a way of giving back to the profession. If specific programs at hospitals allow senior nurses to give back to the system and their profession, those nurses can surely be retained in health care.

Hospital administrators should be creative in designing new roles for senior nurses. Some of the innovative ideas from Robert Wood Johnson's report, *Wisdom at Work: The Importance of the Older and Experienced Nurse in the Workplace* (Hatcher et al., 2006), include senior nurses serving as:

- Mentor for new nurses to help sharpen their skills.

- Preceptors to integrate new nurses into the organization and/or assist with transitions.

- Technology facilitator to incorporate new technology into practice.

- Team builder to coach nurses and physicians in corrective approaches.

- Community liaison to improve public relations.

- Relief nurse to provide patient care when clinical nurses are off duty.

- Safety officer to recommend preventive patient care.

- Staff developer to address professional development issues.

- Patient educator for patients and their families.

- Family advocate to help patients and family negotiate the care delivery system.

- Quality coach to use data for evidence-based practice to improve patient care.

This list should spark much creative thinking to help senior nurses find new ways to provide valuable service in the hospital, drawing upon their skills and experience to design work appropriate to their stage in life.

The research about senior nurses supports what nurses themselves have said over and over: that they could and would like to fill the role of mentor. While mentoring is promoted in many hospitals, it is often an add-on to regular duties, something an experienced nurse can do for a younger nurse on a volunteer basis when it fits into his or her schedule. But Scripps Health in La Jolla, California, has a distinctive, full-blown mentoring program especially appropriate for senior nurses. Its Clinical Mentor Program includes nurses, most of whom are older than 50, with a proven track record as experts at the bedside. These nurses receive an intensive week's orientation with ongoing monthly education. This is an entirely new role, where they no longer practice direct care at the bedside. Instead, they monitor patients and work as coaches to other nurses to improve patient care and teamwork. Clinical mentors are part of patient care every day on every shift. The nurses chosen are highly satisfied with their new roles, so they are remaining in the hospital. Clinical mentoring has become so popular that 59 nurses out of 800 are mentors. How can the hospital afford this kind of change? It was estimated that if they could make at least a 10% improvement in patient outcomes, the savings would pay for clinical mentors. The changes have surpassed expectations. This unique program represents an attractive, innovative way to retain nurses and improve patient care, and it gives Third Age nurses something they have asked for: mentoring.

Massachusetts General Hospital in Boston, Massachusetts, has also recently initiated a novel approach in mentoring. A senior nurse at Massachusetts General Hospital has designed a very innovative change for himself and the nursing staff. Ed Coakley, RN, who has been at Massachusetts General Hospital for more than 35 years, has totally changed his work to focus on one specific area. Ten years ago, he left a nurse executive position to return, after a self-sponsored sabbatical, to a new, complex role as clinical nurse, research associate, and program developer. Now in his mid-60s, he has focused on geriatric care. He sensed a disconnect in the system—a growing number of geriatric patients requiring special services with a shrinking number of nurses to care for them. He designed a program that targeted senior nurses. Ed believes senior nurses are generally better attuned to the needs of geriatric patients than younger nurses. His innovative idea, expressed in the Aging Nurse Project, involves bringing together senior and younger nurses in a residency program that educates them about the latest information and research relating to geriatric care.

Coakley won a sizeable grant from Health and Human Services, Health Resources and Services Administration (HRSA) to fund an ongoing development of his project. Each year, 30 nurses participate in the RN residency, "Transitioning to Geriatrics and Palliative Care," as part of their normal clinical workload. They form intergenerational teams that apply their learning and develop appropriate skills to improve the care of a geriatric population. These trained senior nurses also act as mentors to younger nurses. As Coakley explained in several interviews, the Aging Nurse Project is developing a new delivery system by providing better care for geriatric patients and their families. This unique innovation serves several important purposes:

- It improves patient care.

- It provides professional development for nurses.

- It retains senior nurses.

- It creates organizational transformation.

- It inspires and renews senior nurses, which helps keep them in the system.

Now 65, Coakley is still going strong. A task in Third Age Life Planning (see Chapter 1) is to design work to suit the way you want to live; this program is helping senior nurses do that. The Aging Nurse Project illustrates how a clinical nurse can transform his own role and create new roles for both senior and young nurses to improve a critically important area of patient care.

A number of other hospitals have innovative programs for senior nurses. Rush-Copley Medical Center has a program where nurses, in a new role, are in charge of the process of patient flow from admissions to discharge. At Mount Sinai in New York, senior nurses relieve the clinical nurse by helping patients with discharge and adjusting at home. Senior nurses are also becoming members of research teams that are implementing evidence-based practice. At Mercy Health System, senior nurses mentor young nurses. Thus, new positions are beginning to appear in hospitals around the country, especially with the advance of technology. For example, senior nurses experienced in cardiology can assist bedside nurses by monitoring the functioning of patients' hearts using telemetry, without having to walk up and down long corridors.

6. Education, Training, and Leadership Development

As indicated earlier in this chapter, moving into new roles and career paths often requires and is facilitated by formal learning programs. Nearly all of the top-ranked hospitals have made a commitment to support the learning and development of all nurses, especially senior nurses. A spinoff of this commitment is an improvement in retention. It is generally recognized that the more education nurses have, the more satisfied they are with their work and the longer they remain active in nursing. Support for ongoing education and skill development pays big dividends. Yale-New Haven Hospital, with a strong graduate degree-granting nursing school, might be expected to have a commitment to ongoing learning for all its nurses, which it does. Recently, however, it has broken from a tradition of supporting only young nurses in advancing their education by encouraging senior nurses to pursue education. It grants tuition reimbursement and institutional support for nurses who pursue a Bachelor of Science (BSN) degree and/or a Master of Science (MSN) degree. A few experienced nurses who have started a master's program after 50 have advanced to leadership positions within hospitals or gone on to teach nursing at nearby affiliated schools of nursing. So, another new role for senior nurses is to fill teaching positions in degree-granting programs. For those with many years at the bedside, this role is proving to be a very satisfying career transition that retains a senior nurse in the workforce and at the same time meets the need for more nurse faculty.

Mercy Health System, like others in the AARP list, offers a variety of learning and development programs to both full-time and part-time employees with tuition reimbursement, in-house classroom education, online education, and certificate classes. In the past year, 100% of its employees participated in at least one program, with an average of 25 hours spent in education. Employees are also offered opportunities for the development of new skills by working in temporary assignments, team projects, and a formal rotation program.

Scripps Health also demonstrates its commitment to retain senior, experienced nurses by its learning programs. Through its Center for Learning, all employees, including mature nurses seeking new skills, have many opportunities to develop, learn, and grow through a variety of courses and tuition reimbursement. In its "build talent" program, all costs related to the pursuit of an advanced degree are paid by Scripps Health. One current student is 56 years old. Massachusetts General Hospital similarly has 100% of its employees participating, with an average time of 20 hours spent in education. In response to employee requests, the tuition reimbursement program has been expanded to include advanced certification and "steps to success" to support career development changes. As noted previously in this chapter, it also has a residency program for senior nurses to focus on geriatric patient care.

Large, prestigious hospitals, especially those with medical and nursing schools, might be expected to have full-blown learning for all nurses, and they do. However, some less well-known hospitals show an even stronger commitment, providing a variety of learning opportunities and often more time allowed for them. One hundred percent of Scottsdale Healthcare's employees participated in a comprehensive learning program. In addition, all employees receive annual performance appraisals, which guide them in selecting learning programs. Recently an onsite degree program has expanded by more than 50% and now includes a master's degree. And, 98% of Centegra Health System's employees participated in at least one learning program, with an average of 39 hours spent in education. A "Crucial Conversations" program was also designed with16 hours of education to help resolve issues, build stronger relations, and keep patients safe.

In addition, St. Barnabas in West Orange, New Jersey, has multiple learning opportunities in which 90% of its nurses participated last year, with an average of 47 hours spent in education. It has a special program for senior nurses: its Professional Practice Council focuses on retention, aging workforce issues, patient satisfaction, and leadership development. Nurses can also gain new skills by working on temporary assignments, team projects, and a job rotation program.

Trinitas Hospital in Elizabeth, New Jersey, has 100% of its employees engaged in a variety of learning programs, averaging 45 hours for each individual. A "Bridge to Success" program supports the nurses' ongoing development. As more and more nurses older than 50 participate in learning that supports career development, their competence is increased, which opens up new possibilities for them. Thus, they are going to be more inclined to serve in health care beyond retirement age.

7. Retirement Transition

In Chapter 2, we discussed new developments in retirement that redefine it as an ongoing process, a long transition in the Third Age from full employment—a gradual shift of emphasis and time commitment, often within one's place of work. Nurses can be retained in a significant number of positions in health care beyond retirement age if they have the opportunity to design retirement transitions. Several of the outstanding hospitals in the AARP list have already designed their own versions of this idea, with formal phased retirement programs that keep senior nurses engaged for many years past retirement age.

At Massachusetts General Hospital, employees are encouraged to think ahead toward retirement, invest in their 403(b) plan, and receive help with retirement and financial planning from staff members, financial experts, and planning seminars. Senior nurses can also participate in a formal phased retirement program and are eligible to move to part-time work on a permanent or temporary basis with full benefits.

In 2005, a formal phased retirement program was added to its already varied alternative work arrangements at Mercy Health System. Its "Work to Retire" program allows employees older than 50 to work reduced hours, and employees older than 55 with 15 years of service can work 1,000 hours seasonally. Nurses older than 60 find the new phased retirement program allows them to continue in health care with reduced hours, while retaining full benefits. They have various options, such as seasonal work, which allows them to take extended periods of time off; reduced hours in a regular year's schedule; or job sharing, where two people occupy one full-time position. In addition to fewer hours, nurses can also fill roles that are less physically demanding. About 5% of its nurses have enrolled in this program. The gain for Mercy Health System is more nursing hours from its pool of 96 retirees, who can take temporary work assignments, consulting, or contract work. Because 95% of employees report high satisfaction with their work, the nurses in retirement transition are likely to continue to serve well into their 60s and beyond.

Several other small- or mid-sized hospitals also have their own variations of this program. Nurses at St. John Health in Warren, Michigan, are assisted in preparing for retirement. They are encouraged to invest in a 403(b) plan that allows those older than 50 to make catch-up contributions. Onsite certified retirement representatives assist in pension and retirement planning. Now a phased retirement program allows full-time employees to move into reduced hours as they approach planned retirement. Those who retire can also return to work on a part-time basis and receive full pension benefits.

West Virginia University Hospital has multiple incentives for those interested in phasing into retirement. Nurses have options in flex scheduling, per diem work or weekends only, job sharing, and moving to part-time status on a temporary or permanent status. If they work at least 20 hours per week, they retain full benefits. They may also attend seminars on retirement planning, elder care, and work-life balance. Likewise, Integra Health System has a program that helps employees prepare for retirement; the program includes financial planning from staff and external experts, with special service designed for those over 50 and their spouses. Within its alternative work schedules, a formal, phased retirement program allows full-time nurses the opportunity to move to part-time status on a temporary or permanent basis. Pinnacle Health System in Harrisburg, Pennyslvania, has a phased retirement program that includes that an option for employees approaching retirement to work on a part-time status with no more than 16 hours and still retain full benefits. Like the other hospitals, this program also has financial and retirement planning services for nurses and other employees.

Retirement transition is particularly appropriate for Third Age nurses, and we expect programs that are uniquely suited to their situations will be available at more hospitals. Some hospital administrators, like Scripps Health, have begun to formulate a staged retirement, allowing employees older than 55 who have worked at least 1,000 hours in the past 3 years to continue working half-time with full benefits. But the evolution of this significant new option proposed in Chapter 2 requires a concerted effort from hospital and pension administrators and Third Age Life Coaches to help senior nurses design a long transition that is personally fulfilling and beneficial to quality patient care.

8. Recruitment of Senior Nurses

Some hospital administrators have encouraged mature workers, even those over 50, to consider a career in nursing. With a life expectancy stretching into the 80s, 90s, or even longer, more people are planning for Third Age Careers. Some are designing their own retirement transition, taking courses toward an RN license at a local university or community college to qualify for employment as a nurse. A few hospitals in the AARP list of Best Employers for Workers Over 50 have advertisements stating they seek mature, experienced employees. Some administrators, like those at Scripps Health, have encouraged mature employees in their system to change careers as part of a Life Cycle Employment program. In 2007, 1,128 employees transferred from their current jobs to other positions in the system, based on what they wanted from work and their careers. Twenty-three percent of these people were 50 or older. The career transitions of Third Age nurses represent one way to expand the nurse workforce.

Another option with even more potential is to tap the pool of retirees. Although focused interviews with senior nurses in California did not find much, if any, interest among retirees in returning to nurse work, some facilities have had success with this option. Staff at West Virginia University Hospital stay in touch with the retirees and offer them temporary, part-time, and even full-time work if they want it. Nurses who have been out of the workforce and want to return can take a two-week refresher course and then work in the hospital. At Lee Memorial Health System in Fort Myers, Florida, $1,000 is offered as reimbursement for books and tuition for those enrolled in their nurse refresher program. Yale-New Haven Hospital also has a refresher program of 18 classes, which meet weekdays from 8:30 a.m. to 3:30 p.m. This program, for nurses older than 50 who have been away from nursing and want to return, has even led some nurses to go on for more education and positions of greater responsibility. Pinnacle Health System maintains an active program for its 1,300 retirees, who can return to work part-time in various ways. Durham Regional Hospital in Durham, North Carolina, has a specific "Return to Work" program for its retirees. Trinitas Hospital has only 60 retirees, but it has an active program with a staff person responsible for retiree relations; retired nurses are offered flexible work schedules on a per diem basis. At St. John Health, an individual is assigned to be directly responsible for retiree relations; nurses can work on a part-time, temporary basis and in volunteer opportunities. Rush-Copley Medical Center and Scottsdale Healthcare have similar programs for their retired nurses.

These efforts scattered around the country in many different kinds of hospitals confirm that some nurses are already experiencing the paradox of working retirements. We expect this trend to increase.

9. Support and Recognition

In focused interviews, senior nurses confessed that too often they felt under-appreciated, unrecognized, and unrewarded for their service. Also, they did not receive the kind of support they wanted and needed for personal and professional development.

Administrators at leading hospitals are now taking measures to correct that situation by building a culture of support with special programs and new behaviors. Yale-New Haven Hospital is an outstanding example of how this can be accomplished. Several years ago the senior administration created a culture of support to fulfill its slogan, "Great place to work." We have previously noted how learning programs have been expanded to include senior nurses at Yale-New Haven and a few other hospitals, providing them support for their career development and professional growth, and an enhanced sense of camaraderie and teamwork. Another innovation to build a team environment and shared governance has been "rounding," a program copying the regular physician-patient visitation of "rounds." At Yale-New Haven,

executives and managers have a formal program of rounding, whereby they interact on a one-to-one basis with all their direct reports.
It is more than just a variation of management by walking around
(MBWA) pioneered by Hewlett Packard. This frequent, personal in-
teraction builds open communication, trust, a greater sense of shared
governance, and friendly relationships. Nurses have been involved in
all aspects of building a distinctive organizational culture at Yale-New
Haven. It is no surprise to learn that more than 100 nurses older than
60 work there, and several are older than 70.

Several hospitals also have new programs especially for those over
50. Lee Memorial Health System has a program that targets senior
employees with SHARE (Seniors Health Activities Resource Education), a free club offering health screenings, luncheons, cafeteria and
gift shop discounts, a computer learning center, and social activities.
Mercy Health System has a Senior Connection program for those older than 55 that arranges senior activities and provides assistance with
everyday tasks such as dry cleaning, film development, car care, and
reservations. Massachusetts General Hospital has a host of programs
for older workers, including eldercare discussions, "single again"
financial seminars, grief programs, child care for grandchildren, and
paid leave for family care.

Many hospital administrators have also made a commitment to
show appreciation to nurses for outstanding service with a variety of
recognition programs. Several years ago, as it was building a supportive culture, the senior staff at Yale-New Haven initiated several award
programs to find and honor its finest nurses. In 2007, five of its nurses
were honored with nurse leadership awards. In the same year, 12 more
of its nurses were nominated for the Nightingale Award, an honor
recognizing nurses' commitment to excellence in nursing practice. Of
16 employees named for the "I am Yale-New Haven Service Excellence Heroes" award, five were nurses. In 1991, Yale-New Haven built

a ladder called the Clinical Advancement Program, with three rungs. In 2007, 37 nurses were recognized in quarterly ceremonies for reaching the prestigious level of Clinical Nurse III, and 137 were recognized for attaining Clinical Nurse II. Each year, Yale-New Haven takes the opportunity to recognize outstanding nurse service during National Nurses Week; in 2007, 67 of them were recognized as Nurse of the Year. Clearly nurses at Yale-New Haven feel honored, supported, and recognized for their valuable service.

Mercy Health System is another hospital where building a supportive culture is important. It also has a distinctive recognition program, called ABCD (Above and Beyond the Call of Duty). Along with other employees, nurses who have been "caught" providing exceptional service are recognized with a letter, picture on the wall, special activities, including a luncheon, and a share in cost savings if their service has contributed to those savings. It does not take much to let nurses know how valued they are for providing excellent services. When honored, recognized, and rewarded for service, senior nurses are more likely to stay.

> "When honored, recognized, and rewarded for service, senior nurses are more likely to stay."

10. Succession Planning

Business executives have increasingly realized that a major threat to their company's continued success and vitality is the potential loss of expert knowledge, wisdom, skill base, and strategically important connections that can occur when key people leave before adequately preparing successors. Many of even the most astute and competent organizational leaders have discovered after retirement that they did not invest enough of themselves in preparing people who are expected to follow them. Professor David Garvin, an expert in learning organizations, has argued that a litmus test of a great company is how much is lost with the departure of key people (Garvin, 2003). Preventing wisdom from walking out the door, especially with an aging workforce, requires concerted, sustained efforts to expand core learning and values throughout the organization. Garvin has laid out a very practical approach to building learning organizations. The vital lessons from learning organizations apply to hospitals facing the crisis of a nurse shortage. The crisis stems not just from having too few nurses, but from the threat of losing many of the most experienced, competent, and knowledgeable professionals engaged in patient care. The challenge is not only to retain these nurses, but also to design a culture that allows them to hand down their wisdom, knowledge, and expertise to the younger generation.

Several areas already covered in this chapter are relevant to succession planning. Hospitals promoting shared governance, such as Scripps Health, have also focused on learning and leadership development, so their senior nurses can guide and foster the development of younger nurses. A key role of leaders is to develop leaders. Leadership is not just a role of the few, but an expanding function of a healthy organization. Mentoring, especially through a carefully designed program such as the Clinical Mentors of Scripps Health, also fosters leadership development across generations. It lays a foundation for succession planning as part of nurse development. Drawing upon the knowledge reservoirs of retired nurses is another way to promote the retention of good sense and know-how in patient care that hospitals cannot afford to lose. Hospital administrators committed to sustained excellence in patient care need to design strategies for effective succession planning that retain senior nurses as leaders in their profession. We find little evidence this area has received the serious attention shown in other strategic areas. Hospital administrators can better prepare for the future if they offer their nurses Third Age Life Planning that encourages them to design a more fulfilling second half of life in which, among other things, they concentrate upon leaving a legacy that gives meaning and purpose to their lives.

11. Wellness

An obvious but too easily overlooked factor in the retention of nurses is their own health and condition of well-being. A significant part of Third Age Life Planning includes taking good care of yourself. Many people, as they age, have not done that very well. In the new paradigm of positive aging, the conventional aspects of aging (before 75 or 80), such as decline, disease, disability, and disengagement, are replaced with renewal, rejuvenation, engagement, health, and vitality. Hospital administrators and staff can and should provide support to Third Age nurses regarding self-care and encourage them to become actively involved in regimens that promote vital, healthy, active lifestyles. Some have begun wellness programs geared at preventing disease; a few have a more elaborate response.

Most hospitals in the AARP list of Best Employers for Workers Over 50 have basic wellness programs that include flu shots, smoking cessation, health screenings and appraisals, weight loss, stress management training, physical/activity programs, and health club discounts. Lee Memorial Health System has these basic programs, and in addition provides exercise and yoga classes, free access to onsite health centers, and free medication to employees with hypertension, diabetes, and high cholesterol. Massachusetts General Hospital has a full array of wellness programs, with the basic elements plus a "Be Fit Program" that includes personal training, promoting healthy eating and exercise. In a given year, 95% of its employees have participated in at least one of the wellness programs. Scripps Health has a full basic program and offers free onsite massage therapy as well to help employees cope with stress and tension. In addition to a basic wellness program, Mercy Health System provides health club discounts and a Mercy Safety Fair. In 2007, 94% of its employees used at least one program. In addition to a basic program, Trinitas Hospital has seminars and support groups in exercise, eye care, coping with cancer, and cholesterol management.

St. John Health offers a basic wellness program and has lunch and learning programs featuring health topics, walking groups, and health fairs. At Centegra Health System, the basic package of the "Wellness for Life" program helps employees identify and prevent health/disease issues and make healthy choices. In addition to keeping senior nurses actively engaged in their own well-being, these programs are helping the nurses serve as role models to patients regarding wellness care. By sustaining good health, senior nurses are much more likely to remain in the system.

12. Anchor Changes Into the Culture

After making changes designed to retain senior nurses, hospital administrators need to make sure those changes become part of their organizational culture. The 11 strategic areas previously discussed are interrelated like filaments in a web, where movement in one part reverberates in other parts. To keep them alive and mutually supportive of each other, they need to be anchored in the organization's culture. Too often, new elements conflict with old patterns and assumptions. Clarification of what has been changed and why helps people understand and promote the new directions. Designing a coherent culture can bring consistency and build long-term success.

Culture has an inner, invisible side—the heart of a culture contains the organization's vision, mission, and core values. The external part of culture is expressed in actions, policies, rules, and support/reward systems. People bring their culture to life when they have a firm sense of answers to these questions:

- Who are we?

- What do we stand for and value?

- What do we believe in?

> "Too often, new elements conflict with old patterns and assumptions. Clarification of what has been changed and why helps people understand and promote the new directions."

- What's really important?

- Where are we going now?

- How are we expected to do things around here?

The collective design of a culture helps people formulate answers to these guiding questions. When senior nurses believe they are deeply connected to a place that recognizes them as invaluable players and includes them in shaping a caring, supportive culture that aims to excel in patient care, they will be more open to and interested in remaining in service past retirement age.

The previous examples in this chapter make it obvious Scripps Health has excelled in many areas; not surprisingly, the entire workforce has also consciously worked to anchor the changes and improvements in its culture. Several years ago, Scripps asked, "How can we build an environment that is attractive, especially to senior nurses?" Its leaders realized the critical shortage of nurses would have a devastating impact on Scripps Health, because within a few years roughly 40% of its nurses would be older than 50. If the customary retirement pattern had continued, by now they would have run out of nurses to care for patients. They are preventing that from happening by taking innovative, constructive steps in strategic areas. Improvements have become embedded in the new organizational culture.

Yale-New Haven Hospital also provides an example of a place that has been building a culture that sustains many of the strategic areas covered in this chapter. It already had a competitive compensation and benefit package. It allows nurses to modify their schedules, with greater options for reduced hours, while still retaining benefits. Administrators are now considering other options, such as a 20-hour, 4-day week. They have also improved the physical environment for nurses with ergonomic design. Hospital leaders have promoted shared governance, with nurses involved throughout the emerging culture. Nurses have formed an influential Nursing Cabinet, and its Staff Nurse Council plays an active role in governance. Its evidence-based practice is used as a guide for clinical decision-making, and it has developed improved teamwork and patient safety. Not surprisingly, its patient satisfaction scores have soared. Because the hospital is committed to ongoing learning through a variety of educational programs and training, it promotes nurse development and innovation. This emphasis has led to senior nurses taking on new roles as mentors, educators, and in community outreach. With the emergence of shared governance, learning, and development, nurses feel supported, and the variety of award programs makes them feel recognized and honored. A phased retirement program has not yet been initiated, but interest in doing so exists. All of these steps in critically important areas have led to changes that last.

Final Thoughts

The selective examples described in this chapter show how hospital leadership can develop strategies, policies, and practices that support keeping senior nurses active and at the same time improve patient care, often with a side benefit of cost reduction. An enlightened approach to the current nurse shortage crisis recognizes that senior nurses are more likely to remain in the system if they are adequately compensated, have a supportive workplace that also allows them more control over their work and schedules, gives them an active voice in decision-making and environmental design, recognizes their service and accomplishments, provides ongoing learning that leads them to discover varied challenges and opportunities in new roles, looks to them to be responsible for the transfer of knowledge and succession planning, and helps them design a retirement transition that makes working beyond retirement age attractive.

References

AARP (2007). Best employers for workers over 50 program. Retrieved January 27, 2009, from http://www.aarp.org/money/work/best_employers/

Castro, A.B. (Septermber, 2004). Handle with care. *Online Journal of Issues in Nursing*. Vol. 9:3.

Fortune. (February 4, 2008). 100 best companies to work for 2008. *Fortune*.

Garvin, D. (2003). *Learning in action: A guide to putting the learning organization to work*. Cambridge, MA: Harvard Business School Press.

Hatcher, B., Bleich, M. R., Connolly, C., Davis, K., O'Neill, H., and Hill, K. S. (2006). (Eds.) *Wisdom at work: The importance of the older and experienced nurse in the workplace*. Princeton, NJ: Robert Wood Johnson Foundation. Retrieved January 27, 2009 from http://www.rwjf.org/files/publications/other/wisdomatwork.pdf

Hospitals & Health Networks (January 2008). Chicago: Magazine published by American Hospital Association.

Kotter, J. (1996). *Leading Change*. Cambridge, MA: Harvard Business School Press.

Robert Wood Johnson Foundation. (2008, April). *Charting nursing's future*. Princeton, NJ: Author. Retrieved January 27, 2009, from http://www.rwjf.org/humancapital/index.jsp.

U.S. News & World Report. (July 10, 2008). Best hospitals honor roll. *U.S. News & World Report*. Retrieved January 27, 2009 from http://health.usnews.com/articles/health/best-hospitals/2008/07/10/best-hospitals-honor-roll.html

Working Mother. (2008). 100 best companies. Retrieved January 27, 2009 from http://www.workingmother.com/?service=vpage/109

Creating Tomorrow's 7
Nurse Workforce

This book began with a call to action. To address the critical shortage of nurses at the beginning of the 21st century, we proposed focusing on retaining senior nurses in the health care system beyond retirement age, in addition to expanding recruitment of new nurses in institutions of higher learning. However, in the process of research, consultation, and writing, our initially conceived tactic has taken on a larger, unexpected perspective. We have learned directly from nurses themselves, as well as from other research, reports, and analyses, that the development of senior nurses to meet the crisis also indicates a need for a grand strategy to advance the professional development of senior nurses to improve the quality of patient care, contribute to the strength and viability of a national health care system, reduce health care costs, and set new models for a more productive retirement. The call to action has led to a new vision of and mission for nurses in the Third Age. The dire prospect of a huge shortage of nurses and the need for a more productive and inclusive health care system have the potential to vitally transform nurse careers and health care.

A New Vision/Mission for Third Age Nurses

We find several reasons for a new vision.

"The dire prospect of a huge shortage of nurses and the need for a more productive and inclusive health care system has within it the potential for a vital transformation of nurse careers and health care."

- First, the dramatic changes in the life course have not only significantly stretched life expectancy for healthy individuals, but many people, including nurses, are demonstrating *vital* capacities for productivity, creativity, leadership, and community service decades beyond the usual retirement age. Furthermore, baby boomers, including nurses, who have already started to turn 60, have indicated a strong desire to continue working (Miller, 2008).

- Second, the conventional notion of retirement has been changing fast, with most senior Americans already experiencing the paradox of "working retirement." This shift can produce a serendipity effect, as many companies, including health care organizations, threatened with a loss of key people they can't afford to let go, realize an unanticipated opportunity to retain the employees with knowledge, wisdom, experience, skills, commitment, and connections that are vital to organizational effectiveness and success.

- Third, a few health care organizations have already been creatively changing the way nurses experience and provide service; there are models of how health care organizations and nurses can collaborate to build new models of development and productivity.

An analysis of the emerging demographic, social, and organizational situations has led to a vision of a nurse professional whose career extends far beyond the common retirement age of late 50s or early 60s. As senior nurses engage in Third Age Life Planning, they tap their potential for ongoing personal renewal and professional development, which contributes to new models for better patient care; improved health care collaboration; mentoring of new nurses; and valuable, sustained input into health care systems. Nurses can now view their professional career as a series of developments, accompanied by continued learning and new experiences, that build new forms of leadership. These developments leave a legacy of meaning for themselves, their colleagues, and those they serve. As their careers move through a long retirement transition, they will have opportunities for a greater balance of life and work, of personal time with professional service, and of individual passion with social contribution. However, for this vision to become a vibrant reality, individual nurses, communities of nurses, and their employers must join together to forge a new pathway into the future of health care. New careers for Third Age nurses promise greater fulfillment to individual nurses and set a standard for other professions to follow. That is an exciting vision of new pathways in nursing careers.

Needed Action by Third Age Nurses

For this change to happen, action must initiate with those who want the change—the Third Age nurses—and it must occur as a group effort if anything is to change. This reality means nurses must join together, either through established organizations or as a new effort, to energize the interest and untapped desires of Third Age nurses to change the way care is delivered to the public.

Throughout this book, the message has been consistent and vital: Third Age nurses want to continue to serve the public because they love nursing, but want to do so in a different way. We cannot afford to lose the skills and expertise of Third Age nurses. However, to expect others to initiate and carry forth this needed change is both naïve and improbable. So how will this large and unfulfilled group of nurses

"Nurses can now view their professional career as a series of developments, accompanied by continued learning and new experiences, building toward new forms of leadership that leave a legacy of meaning for themselves, their colleagues, and those they serve."

generate the needed actions to promote their inclusion in the workforce of the future? This book has explored many ways this can be accomplished by individuals and organizations, but the answer to this question actually belongs to those who want to see the change and are willing to exert the effort.

As is the case with change in any form, individual, group, and political aspects must be addressed before any movement can take place. In other words, you have to get the ducks lined up before the march can begin. Third Age nurses need to complete a self-assessment to determine what they really want in the future and what they can offer to make any change occur. In this book, we have offered many options to help nurses do this assessment. We have also suggested many ways the Third Age nurse can prepare for workforce re-entry and/or a shift in activity. But this is the easy aspect of change; the next step is to get the support and inclusion of other nurses, so that together they can be available to address what needs to change.

Nurses throughout history have been the "movers and shakers" for change in health care. It all began with Florence Nightingale, the founder of modern nursing. Given her position as a wealthy woman in England, she was able to convert the way injured soldiers were treated during the Crimean War, which made a major impact on the treatment of the sick public throughout the world. Her insistence on a clean environment changed the way health care was delivered then and is in the forefront today as a way to avoid infections and to promote healthy lifestyles.

Many others have also left a legacy as models for change, such as Clara Barton, the founder of the American Red Cross, and Lillian Wald, who established the New York City Henry Street Settlement, the first visiting nurse service in the United States. In addition, Margaret Sanger founded the American Birth Control League, which eventually became Planned Parenthood (after she served some jail time to accomplish this goal). And, Mary Breckinridge founded the Frontier Nursing Service, where nurses provided care on horseback to rural areas of Kentucky. Many other nurses have devoted their lives to the betterment of humankind in the form of better health care. However, they all had one thing in common—they were devoted to a cause and willing to do whatever it took to reach their goals. They persevered in times when women were not recognized as leaders and when a need for change existed.

Given these women as good role models, Third Age nurses can do the same. They can move forward into a system that is begging for change by making clear that there are ways to accomplish change. They can do this alone or as a group, but they must consider the obstacles and the facilitators before they move forward, just as their predecessors in change did. Florence Nightingale knew her facilitators and the obstacles. She knew her father's position and wealth gave her an edge. She also knew a woman at the battlefront was unheard of. But, she balanced these obstacles against her facilitators and made major changes in health care throughout the world. It was not easy, but she persisted.

The same is true of the other nurses who initiated change. They all knew the dangers of making change, but they acted carefully, balancing the positives against the negatives. Sanger had to pay for the activities in some form, but she was willing to do so even if it meant spending time in jail. Sanger was adamant about her cause and had a history of persistence like never before seen. To the day she died, at 87 years old, she was publishing articles and traveling throughout the world, lecturing and helping to establish clinics for women interested in birth control. She died in 1966, only a few months after the *Griswold v. Connecticut* decision, which legalized birth control for married couples in the United States, the apex of her 50-year career (Lewis, n.d.).

Getting Started

In contrast to how it was in the past, nurses cannot start this journey for change alone. They face too many obstacles, particularly in the U.S. health care system, even though it desperately needs to be changed. The obstacle/facilitator ratio leans *too* much toward the obstacles and not enough toward the facilitators. Even though everyone knows the system needs to change, the change agent must be powerful and interested in the change, and that means looking for appropriate help. Third Age nurses need to be part of a major movement initiated by a large and politically astute organization, such as the American Nurses Association. With a membership of hundreds of thousands, that organization finds it easy to be heard. And because its mission is to be the spokesperson for nurses, this organization is one to consider. The same is true of the many specialty organizations, such as AARP. This organization has a history of advocating for the elderly and for programs that assist the aged. It has also provided help regarding changes for the Third Age nurses. Investigate information from organizations such as Nurse Connect (www.nurseconnect.com) or Secure Path (www.securepathbytransamerica.com), and take the initiative to call their headquarters to voice your questions, concerns, and suggestions for building these new pathways for senior nurses.

Further, as described in Chapter 6 of this book, many hospitals and health care organizations are already being changed. So, a second option is to contact them to see what they are offering. Taking the time to find out about the changes going on in hospitals across the nation and knowing the political issues that support or block these changes are important and necessary steps. This means Third Age nurses need to read, search for, and keep abreast of what is happening. Nurses generally have not been politically attuned, up-to-date, or even interested in the issues being discussed and the options being made available for older nurses. They often do not even know how to find out what is available and happening. As Sally Power (n.d.) has written, nurses need to build bridges and stay connected.

Being a member of a nurse organization that provides current information and an option to suggest topics for discussion provides Third Age nurses with quick and easy access to the world of health care information. Going back to school to acquire an advanced degree can do the same thing and probably at a greater depth. Success today demands nurses know what is happening in health care and what should occur to improve access and reduce cost. Courses in economics and health care ethics provide valuable knowledge that every nurse should have and are offered by most nursing programs in the United States. Also, everything needed as a basis for quality nursing practice is not always offered within nursing programs, so investigate what is available in business, sociology, and psychology programs to stay current and employable. Another great resource is the book *Opportunities to Care: The Pfizer Guide to Careers in Nursing* (2002).

Creating a New Pathway

One message we've tried to convey in this book is to create a Third Age Life Portfolio, which means thinking about the next step in a career as part of a pathway. This is true regarding the selection of a new position rather than retirement or the return from retirement. As Tamara Erickson states in her 2008 book *Retire Retirement,* it is time to think ahead. Think about how the next experience and new position will fit into the pathway; the decision of "what's next" should not be put off for a few years. Building a life portfolio requires imagining and thinking beyond the next option.

A review of the lives of our historical nurse heroes indicates they had one overarching interest. They had several jobs and positions, but they were all related. Florence Nightingale established many programs and helped many nurses, but she always had her sights set on quality care. Our other historical nurses did the same thing. They had a mission, and they did what was necessary to keep that mission alive and functioning. Today, Third Age nurses can pick a direction or a specialty and move from job to job or from activity to activity within that specialty, so that when one option is too demanding or too boring, another option opens up.

Third Age nurses cannot sit by and be silent, nor can they expect others to speak for them. They must believe they are an important and valuable asset to the health care system and that they are needed, and not only because of a nurse shortage. They have the experience within a rapidly changing health care system, having seen the incredible change, and thus have demonstrated they can adjust to and initiate change. Newly graduated nurses might be up-to-date, but they have not had the experience of making change or of knowing what needs to change.

The development of evidence-based practice, SBAR communication (where nurses describe the situation, background, and make an assessment and recommendations to the physician), family-centered care, and many other innovations have been introduced and implemented by Third Age nurses. The electronic medical record and the use of robots in surgery were possible only because nurses in the workforce during the past decades joined with other health care professionals in these adventures into the future. To lose these nurses to retirement would not only hurt the health care system, but it would also be a great loss for the nurses. Such innovations are just the beginning of what we are going to see in the future, and we need a workforce that knows how to introduce and manage change. Third Age nurses know just what is needed and can lead others (the new nurses) forward based on their willingness and experiences with some of the greatest changes in health care in the history of the human race.

So, how can Third Age nurses lead the needed changes? The answer is, just like they did in the past. Using six strategies for change, they can:

1. Stay engaged

2. Keep current

3. Be unafraid

4. Communicate ideas

5. Be creative

6. Take the lead

Stay Engaged

Staying engaged is the most important endeavor Third Age nurses must pursue. Whereas nurses might have a tendency to look forward to retirement, most nurses who have retired are now back in the workforce doing important and different things. For example, it is common to hear from nurses who attempted retirement, but who returned to nursing after they had a little rest, that they were ready for something new and different. Jane, a nurse, told the story of her adventures with retirement when she was interviewed for this book. She had waited anxiously for the day when she could stay in bed in the morning and not have to worry about staffing or any of the other aspects of her manager role. However, that did not last long. She then tried volunteer work with the Red Cross. While that kept her very busy and was rewarding, she kept wondering about the hospital she had left and those whom she had worked with over the last 30 years. She kept weekly lunch dates with her former colleagues so she could keep in touch, but after 3 months of "lunching" she admitted that she really missed caring for patients too.

Her next endeavor was as a public health nurse. Again, she loved the contact with patients and their families in the home, but she was always interested in her former colleagues' activities. At this time she was meeting with them once a month for dinner and getting the up-to-date stories about what they were doing. She was fascinated by their activities and decided to accept an offer to volunteer at the hospital as a mentor for new graduates. This position came to her as a surprise. One of her colleagues offered her name to the hospital chief nurse executive when she heard they were initiating a new mentor program. Being back in her old environment was a great experience, but mentoring as a volunteer was using up a lot of her time and offered no compensation.

Jane's next attempt to take care of her longing for patient care occurred while she was doing some consultation at another hospital that had heard about her activities as a mentor of new graduates. Before long, she was very busy going from one hospital to another helping each initiate mentoring programs. One day she simply stopped and asked herself: "What am I doing? I retired, and now I am working harder then ever and not making the salary I could if I returned to bedside nursing." While she was very engaged and feeling satisfied, she still missed the position she had held for so many years. As Marc Freedman (2007) suggests in his book *Encore*, finding work that matters in the second half of life is important.

Retirement is not what it used to be. It's not easy to stop nurse work, especially if patient contact and being part of health restoration is what you find rewarding. Jane is 70 years old today and is still providing bedside care. She is the first to admit she enjoyed all of the other positions she held, but for her, hospital care is what "turns her on."

Keep Current

Keeping current is another way, as described earlier in this chapter, to stay engaged. But it is also a way to "take the lead." Nurses that keep current can evaluate what is happening to determine if it is in the best interest of the public and if the public is receiving the best preventive information and health care. Keeping current means knowing what is happening in health care, what is a problem, and what is being proposed. For example, the public has been given a great deal of misinformation about medications and immunizations, so they are likely to make incorrect assumptions followed by faulty actions. Several years ago a study by two physicians was published in a renowned professional journal about the implied connection between measles immunizations for infants and the incidence of autism. After national hysteria and hundreds of parents refusing to immunize their children, the study was found to have major limitations; thus, the results were not valid. Although many community and acute care nurses worked hard to reverse these misconceptions, even today some parents are afraid to immunize their children because of this event.

The same possibilities can occur if Third Age nurses do not stay informed about the opportunities, or lack of opportunities, available for them in the workplace so they can take action. Nurses cannot just sit by and accept what they hear. They must, as their predecessors did, keep informed and get involved in seeing things change for the betterment of everyone.

But how do nurses keep informed? Joining a professional group is one excellent way to stay in touch with health care change. Reading professional journals is another. Volunteering at a hospital, a community health care project, or a school can also provide Third Age nurses with valid and important information. Joining the PTA, AARP, or other local, state, or national organizations can provide contact with public activities. The Web is another very rich resource, because a tremendous amount of information can be found online. Even the daily newspaper is a good source of highlighted problems of the public's health. The objective is to seek information, and then to have a source for checking the validity of the information because some of what is gathered online or read in the paper is not always accurate. Still, at least nurses who consult the Web or the newspaper have obtained information, which is better than being without any.

Be Unafraid

Being afraid is an excellent way of isolating yourself from what's going on. Fear is a powerful barrier to interactions, access to information, and currency. Many people isolate themselves from others for fear of "doing the wrong thing," "saying the wrong thing," or because they feel "out of touch." If nurses are engaged and up-to-date, they need not be afraid of doing or saying the wrong thing. In fact, by being engaged and current, Third Age nurses have the tools that foster confidence, which means being ready to take the lead when necessary.

Being afraid commonly leads to not having a positive self-image. Because most nurses are women, and women have been a suppressed population historically and classified as handmaidens to physicians, it is not uncommon for Third Age nurses to have low self-esteem. For example, nurses still act on the orders written by the physician and need to call for permission to alter those orders, despite many facilities considering the plan of care, written by the physician, as the joint effort of both the physician and the nurse. This simple use of words often makes nurses afraid to act independently when making decisions about the patient's care. It tends to create a feeling of not being honored for their intelligence and rights under the laws regarding licensed caregivers.

Getting beyond these fears demands Third Age nurses recognize the value of nursing and the role nurses play in the care of patients. The leaders of nursing, those of the past and those currently in the lead, were not afraid of those in their path. They were more concerned with making the lives of others better and were willing to do so even under the worst circumstances. That is what we need to do today, surge forward knowing the outcome is more important than the feelings of the leader. We must override fear with the desire to make things better. One proven way to overcome fear and clarify your own desired course of development is to engage in Third Age Life Planning with the help of a Life Coach, as suggested in Chapter 1 (See Appendix A for a list of Life Coaches). You also need to be a self-advocate. According to Diane Scott in her 2008 book, *Being a Self-Advocate for Your Professional Life,* becoming a self-advocate "will help guide insight to the path that you must take to triumph over inevitable changes and be happy with your professional and personal choices" (p. 18).

> "The leaders of nursing, those of the past and those currently in the lead, were not afraid of those in their path."

Communicate Ideas

To stay engaged, keep current, and override fear, nurses need to communicate with others to determine the value of and barriers to ideas. Functioning alone can be dangerous because we all need validation, correction, and assurance. Here is where being engaged is important, because engagement provides opportunities for reflection. A friend, colleague, Life Coach, family member, or a group of people can be valuable to help you determine if an idea is worth action and if the outcome of the action is appropriate or possible.

Again, you need to stay connected by being part of an organization such as the American Nurses Association (ANA) that has a huge membership and a powerful voice. If Third Age nurses are to make the needed changes in health care, they need to hear from the membership about the problems and the potential solutions. Third Age nurses can then let the leadership of ANA know what needs to occur so strategies can be devised for change. Also local organizations can be formed, which can be another powerful way to promote engagement, learning, and communication. Third Age nurses should band together to form new ways to support each other, communicate and learn together, and build their own coalitions that can promote the kinds of change they believe are necessary. This book has reported on one example: The Center for Third Age Nurses at Holy Names University in Oakland, California, which has been formed by nurses who inspired each other with a common vision to support the development of senior nurses. At first the Center had no available funds, but nurses found time in their busy schedules to meet, learn together, develop networks of communication, brainstorm ideas, and plan informal activities that reached an expanding circle of like-minded professionals. Eventually, they obtained modest funding to allow planning and organizational formation, which has led to experiments to enlighten, sustain, and develop Third Age nurses. This local innovation should inspire nurses in other regions to build their own local groups to inspire new kinds of learning, leadership, and communication that can improve health care with the professional development and retention of senior nurses.

Until recently, we have not known about the problems and challenges faced by Third Age nurses. Surveys, research, and recent articles have begun to identify the desires, concerns, and needs of these nurses. Still more is needed, so Third Age nurses should communicate in as many ways as possible exactly what they need, want, and can do.

Be Creative

Communication can take many forms. Voice, written words, and actions are the usual ways of forwarding information. Third Age nurses need to develop these and also find other ways of informing the health care systems about their needs, wants, and abilities. For example, artwork in the form of fliers or posters can be circulated by e-mail blasts, which cost nothing for the sender. Presentations can be given at meetings or for groups to provide Third Age information to others. Additionally, Third Age nurses might need to supplement the quiet approach with more assertive, creative actions, such as frequent visits to the chief nurse, or the CEO and board of directors of the hospital.

Being creative means using all of the available means of getting heard, which again might mean joining an organization and getting on a committee. Being heard, being involved, and being persistent are important if change is to occur. Nurse leaders of the past were not silent. Florence Nightingale took on the government of England when she spoke; Lillian Wald did the same when she took on the task of helping the poor; and Clara Barton and Margaret Sanger were both very vocal (Allender & Spradley, 2005). They also worked hard as role models by practicing what they preached; Third Age nurses need to do the same. Seeing is believing and helps to make the talk concrete. Third Age nurses who are creating new roles need to come forward and tell the world about their activities. Putting activities online so others can see what it is like to be involved can also help others understand the new roles.

Take the Lead

The tactics just discussed—staying engaged, keeping current, being unafraid, communicating ideas, and being creative—all lead Third Age nurses to take charge as leaders. Our vision includes the emergence of Third Age nurses as creative, productive leaders of change in the health care system. So, Third Age nurses cannot sit by and wonder about the future or make decisions that lead to unhappiness, discontent, or depression. They need to be active, speak up, and charge forward to determine new pathways instead of taking an early, conventional retirement. As described in Chapter 2, retirement today is being redefined. It is a journey, not a destination. The journey is one that can include a transition with renewal, learning, and discovery. It

"Our vision includes the emergence of Third Age nurses as creative, productive leaders of change in the health care system."

can include different forms of work and a greater balance of personal growth and productivity, which can leave a legacy that adds value to communities, professions, and society. The Third Age for nurses should become a time of redefinition of work and retirement not only for personal fulfillment and professional growth, but for leadership development.

As we described in Chapter 6, Third Age nurses have been taking on leadership roles in countless hospital innovations and cultural changes to improve patient care and to support their own retention and development. Nurse executives, managers, and clinical nurses have teamed up to lead change. They have initiated and supported organizational surveys and reported findings that call for change in policies and practices. They have led the way by introducing the ways nurses can manage their time, activities, and responsibilities with flexible schedules, ergonomics, new technologies, new patterns of career development in retirement transitions, and the design of new roles for improved patient care. In some cases—this number should increase exponentially—nurses have contributed to changes in hospital governance and succession management, which provides opportunities for shared leadership in planning, decision-making, evidence-based practice, team building, and new modalities in improved patient care. In short, hospitals on the cutting edge have benefited greatly from Third Age nurses who have been taking the leadership for change.

In addition to organizational and cultural change, in Chapter 6 we cited numerous examples of clinical nurses who created impressive innovations in both patient care and in nursing practice. Nurse managers have teamed with clinical nurses in research that has led to insights and improved practices in the growth of evidence-based practice. A former executive nurse returned to the bedside and designed a residency program for senior nurses to learn and practice better geriatric care, which involved teams of experienced nurses mentoring younger nurses. In another situation, clinical nurses designed an entirely new role of clinical mentoring, where senior nurses supervised, coordinated, and modeled best practices that have greatly improved patient care, significantly raised patient satisfaction, and lowered costs. Nurses have built stronger internal networks, promoting ongoing learning, expanding excellence, and regenerating recognition for outstanding service. By taking the lead in their hospitals, Third Age nurses have been creating new roles as mentors, educators, facilitators, communicators, patient advocates, and liaisons among health care organizations, patient families, and communities. These few examples point the way to a transformation, not just in professional development but in the nation's health care system.

Taking the lead also means Third Age nurses need to be heard, seen, and valued, which can happen only if they are willing to come forward, get involved, and take a chance. Many have done so, but we do not read about them or see them in the movies or in the popular literature. So another way to take the lead is to write and promote stories in the papers, in the popular literature, and in the professional publications about what Third Age nurses are doing. Reading about a nurse's activities might give other nurses the courage to try the same or to attempt something they are afraid to do.

Final Word

We are on the frontier of another new development in health care, with nurses once again taking the lead. The bottom line comprises involvement, visibility, and new forms of leadership, especially by Third Age nurses. Historically, any cause that created change was generated by those who made themselves heard and seen. Third Age nurses must generate attention for their cause.

This book has shown how some nurses and health care organizations have begun to fashion new pathways for nurses' Third Age Careers. But the movement has just begun. Hopefully, this book will excite, instruct, and motivate many nurses and health care administrators to move forward for significant improvement in health and patient care.

References

Allender, J. A., and Spradley, B. W. (2004). *Community health nursing: Promoting and protecting the public's health*. Philadelphia: Lippincott Williams & Wilkins.

Erickson, T. (2008). *Retire retirement*. Boston: Harvard Business School Press.

Freedman, M. (2007). *Encore: Finding work that matters in the second half of life*. San Francisco: Public Affairs.

Lewis, J. J. (n.d.). Margaret Sanger. Retrieved October 5, 2008, from http://womenshistory.about.com/od/sangermargaret/p/margaret.sanger.htm

Miller, M. (2008). *Retire smart*. Retrieved January 27, 2009, from http://www.securepathbytransamerica.com/app/articleRetireSmart.htm

Pfizer. (2002). *Opportunities to care: The Pfizer guide to careers in nursing*. New York: Pfizer Pharmaceuticals Group.

Power, S. (n. d.). Build your bridge: Second careers. SecurePath. Retrieved January 27, 2009, from http://www.securepathbytransamerica.com/app/articleBuildYourBridge.htm

Scott, D. (2007). Being a self-advocate for your professional life. *South Carolina Nurse*: 14(1), 20.

Coaches for Third Age Life Planning | **A**

There are more than 60,000 members of the International Coaching Federation; a few of them have developed skills for Third Age Life Planning. Leaders in the network of Third Age Life Planning who are especially attuned to the needs of Third Age nurses include the following people:

Melita DeBellis

Principal, Third Age Coaching Certification with the Center for Third Age Leadership
www.thirdagecenter.com (select coaching list) and
www.turning-point-coaching.com
E: melita@turning-point-coaching.com
Burlington, VT
802-434-6600

Nancy Cosgriff

The Center for Third Age Leadership
E: nancy@thirdagecenter.com
Marine on St. Croix, MN
651-307-5285

Dorian Mintzer, PhD

Boomers and Beyond Coach
Licensed Third Age Coach
www.dorianmintzer.com
E: dorian@dorianmintzer.com
Boston, MA
617-267-0585

Margaret (Meg) L. Newhouse, PhD

Passion and Purpose LifeCrafting
www.lifeplanningnetwork.org
E: m-newhouse@comcast.com
Weston, MA
781-893-4260

Roberta Taylor, MA, RN

www.pathmaking.com
E: rkt@pathmaking.com
781-237-7979

Index

Symbols

A

C

Y-Z

Books Published by the Honor Society of Nursing, Sigma Theta Tau International

Why Retire? Career Strategies for Third Age Nurses, Bower and Sadler, 2009.

B Is for Balance: A Nurse's Guide for Enjoying Life at Work and at Home, Weinstein, 2008.

To Comfort Always: A Nurse's Guide to End-of-Life Care, Norlander, 2008.

Ready, Set, Go Lead! A Primer for Emerging Health Care Leaders, Dickenson-Hazard, 2008.

Words of Wisdom From Pivotal Nurse Leaders, Houser and Player, 2008.

Tales From the Pager Chronicles, Rancour, 2008.

The Nurse's Etiquette Advantage, Pagana, 2008.

NURSE: A World of Care, Jaret, 2008. Published by Emory University and distributed by the Honor Society of Nursing, Sigma Theta Tau International.

Nursing Without Borders: Values, Wisdom, Success Markers, Weinstein and Brooks, 2007.

Synergy: The Unique Relationship Between Nurses and Patients, Curley, 2007.

Conversations With Leaders: Frank Talk From Nurses (and Others) on the Front Lines of Leadership, Hansen-Turton, Sherman, and Ferguson, 2007.

Pivotal Moments in Nursing: Leaders Who Changed the Path of a Profession, Houser and Player, 2004 (Volume I) and 2007 (Volume II).

Daily Miracles: Stories and Practices of Humanity and Excellence in Health Care, Briskin and Boller, 2006.

A Daybook for Nurse Leaders and Mentors. Sigma Theta Tau International, 2006.

The HeART of Nursing: Expressions of Creative Art in Nursing, Second Edition, Wendler, 2005.

Making a Difference: Stories from the Point of Care, Volumes I & II, Hudacek, 2005.

A Daybook for Nurses: Making a Difference Each Day, Hudacek, 2004.

Ordinary People, Extraordinary Lives: The Stories of Nurses, Smeltzer and Vlasses, 2003.

For more information and to order these books from the Honor Society of Nursing, Sigma Theta Tau International, visit the society's Web site at www.nursingsociety.org/publications, or go to www.nursingknowledge.org/stti/books, the Web site of Nursing Knowledge International, the honor society's sales and distribution division. Or, call 1.888.NKI.4.YOU (U.S. and Canada) or +1.317.634.8171 (Outside U.S. and Canada).